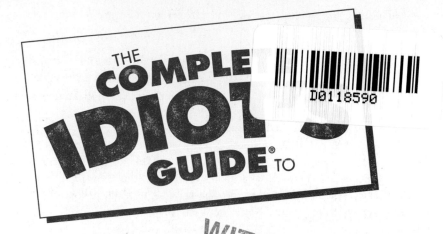

THE COMPLETE IDIOT'S GUIDE® TO

WITHDRAWN

Natural Childbirth

Jennifer L. West, LM, CPM, HBCE,
and Deborah S. Romaine

ALPHA

A member of Penguin Group (USA) Inc.

For expectant mothers everywhere, with joy for your new family

ALPHA BOOKS

Published by the Penguin Group

Penguin Group (USA) Inc., 375 Hudson Street, New York, New York 10014, USA

Penguin Group (Canada), 90 Eglinton Avenue East, Suite 700, Toronto, Ontario M4P 2Y3, Canada (a division of Pearson Penguin Canada Inc.)

Penguin Books Ltd., 80 Strand, London WC2R 0RL, England

Penguin Ireland, 25 St. Stephen's Green, Dublin 2, Ireland (a division of Penguin Books Ltd.)

Penguin Group (Australia), 250 Camberwell Road, Camberwell, Victoria 3124, Australia (a division of Pearson Australia Group Pty. Ltd.)

Penguin Books India Pvt. Ltd., 11 Community Centre, Panchsheel Park, New Delhi—110 017, India

Penguin Group (NZ), 67 Apollo Drive, Rosedale, North Shore, Auckland 1311, New Zealand (a division of Pearson New Zealand Ltd.)

Penguin Books (South Africa) (Pty.) Ltd., 24 Sturdee Avenue, Rosebank, Johannesburg 2196, South Africa

Penguin Books Ltd., Registered Offices: 80 Strand, London WC2R 0RL, England

International Standard Book Number: 978-1-59257-937-2
Library of Congress Catalog Card Number: 2009924929

11 10 09   8 7 6 5 4 3 2 1

Interpretation of the printing code: The rightmost number of the first series of numbers is the year of the book's printing; the rightmost number of the second series of numbers is the number of the book's printing. For example, a printing code of 09-1 shows that the first printing occurred in 2009.

Printed in the United States of America

Note: This publication contains the opinions and ideas of its authors. It is intended to provide helpful and informative material on the subject matter covered. It is sold with the understanding that the authors, book producer, and publisher are not engaged in rendering medical or other professional services in the book. If the reader requires personal assistance or advice, a competent professional should be consulted.

The authors, book producer, and publisher specifically disclaim any responsibility for any liability, loss, or risk, personal or otherwise, which is incurred as a consequence, directly or indirectly, of the use and application of any of the contents of this book.

Most Alpha books are available at special quantity discounts for bulk purchases for sales promotions, premiums, fund-raising, or educational use. Special books, or book excerpts, can also be created to fit specific needs.

For details, write: Special Markets, Alpha Books, 375 Hudson Street, New York, NY 10014.

Publisher: *Marie Butler-Knight*
Editorial Director: *Mike Sanders*
Senior Managing Editor: *Billy Fields*
Executive Editor: *Randy Ladenheim-Gil*
Book Producer: *Lee Ann Chearney/Amaranth IlluminAre*
Development Editor: *Jennifer Bowles*
Senior Production Editor: *Janette Lynn*

Copy Editor: *Lisanne V. Jensen*
Cover Designer: *Kurt Owens*
Book Designer: *Trina Wurst*
Indexer: *Tonya Heard*
Layout: *Brian Massey*
Proofreader: *John Etchison*

Contents at a Glance

Part 1:   **You're Having a Baby, Naturally!**   1

1   Celebrating Your Pregnancy   3
Everyone has a birth story, and now it's your turn to write yours the way you and your baby want to tell it.

2   What Does It Mean to Give Birth Naturally?   13
All that you need to bring a new life into the world you already carry within you. Your woman's body is uniquely designed for this.

3   Weighing the Risks and Rewards   25
Having a natural birth requires planning and preparation. Are you ready for this amazing journey?

Part 2:   **The Truth About Natural Childbirth**   37

4   How Much Will It Hurt … *Really?*   39
For many women, pain is the great unknown with birth. But what if you could birth without pain and without pain medications?

5   Is Your Body in Shape for a Natural Birth?   53
Having a natural birth is one of the most physically intense experiences you could ask of your body. Even though this is what your body's designed to do, there are ways you can prepare.

6   Is a Natural Birth Dangerous?   63
A lot of worry surrounds a natural birth, but do the facts support the fears? (No!)

7   Making a Choice: Midwife or Doctor?   75
Are you ready to do some interviewing? Choosing your practitioner is one of the most important decisions you'll make, and makes the difference for the kind of birth you'll have.

8   Homebirth, Birthing Center, or Hospital?   93
Each has its advantages and drawbacks. Which choice offers the optimal balance for you?

Part 3:   Planning for a Natural Childbirth   107

9   What to Eat   109
Cravings, nutrients, and calories ... oh my! You are what you eat, and so is your baby.

10   Yoga, Stretching, and Massage   119
Your body wants to be strong, flexible, and resilient as it approaches the birth experience. Helping it get and stay that way helps you stay comfortable, too.

11   Preparing for a Mindful Birth   135
Natural birth is the ultimate choreography of your body and mind.

12   Support for Going Natural   147
You're not in this alone. Your birthing team is right there with you to encourage you and to help make sure your birthing is the wonderful experience you've envisioned.

Part 4:   Natural Birthing Methods   159

13   Childbirth Preparation   161
Breathe. Focus. Relax. Learn the many methods you can use to keep your birthing calm and comfortable.

14   Waterbirth   171
Wouldn't it be great to float away your discomforts and welcome your baby into the world gently and fluidly?

15   Birth with Hypnosis   181
Clear the clutter from your mind so you can focus your full effort to work with the natural rhythms of your body.

16   Calling All Doulas   191
A doula can cover all the details you're too busy to bother with once birthing begins, from getting you something to eat to running interference on your behalf.

17   Making Your Birthing Preferences   201
Specific, clear, and in writing: your birthing preferences are the blueprint for the birth you want.

Part 5:   Your Baby's Birthday Arrives!   211

18   Natural Labor   213
Stage by stage, here's what to expect and how to use all the preparation you've worked so hard to put in place.

19 The Nonmedicated Birth   223
*You have a lot of methods available to help you stay
comfortable. Your midwife or doctor, doula, and birthing
team can help you choose the ones likely to be most effective
for you.*

20 What if the Pain Is Too Much … and Other Things
That Can Happen   235
*Sometimes things don't go quite according to plan. But not
to worry … you've considered the possibilities, and you have
a plan in place for them, too.*

Part 6:   **Welcoming Your New Baby**   **249**

21 Your Baby's First Moments, Naturally   251
*How amazing to finally meet this new person! Your baby is
calm, alert, and eager to meet you, too.*

22 Postpartum: What You'll Feel Like   261
*One journey is over, but another is just beginning. From
getting underway with breastfeeding to managing your
rapidly shifting hormones, the first few weeks after your
baby's birth can be intense.*

23 Breastfeeding, of Course   273
*Mother's milk is baby's best food for nutrition as well as
for a healthy immune system, not to mention the bonding
between you and your baby that takes place when your baby
is at your breast.*

24 You'd Do It All Again   283
*How great that you've had a birthing experience you want
to repeat!*

Appendixes

A Resources   291

B Glossary   297

Index   301

Contents

Part I: You're Having a Baby, Naturally!   1

1   Celebrating Your Pregnancy   3

The Birth Story...4

I Had a Great Birth, and Everyone Hates Me!............................5

    Inside the Birth Myths...*6*

    Write Your Own Birth Story..*8*

Reclaiming Birth...8

Giving Yourself the Best Preparation 9

Everything You Need Is Already Within You..........................10

    You Have More Choices Than You Think...............................*10*

Take the Lead!...11

2   What Does It Mean to Give Birth Naturally?   13

Who's in Charge? You! 14

    It's About You, Too *15*

    But I'm Not Really the "Earth-Mother" Type *15*

What a Natural Birth Is *Not*..16

The Winding Road of Birth Intervention 17

    Sleep Tight...*17*

    What Did Caesar Have to Do with It? *19*

    The Regulation of Birth...*20*

Same Goal, Divergent Paths...20

Birth Works...20

    No Place Like Home *21*

    No Hurry..*21*

    The Intervention Cascade...*22*

    Is C-Section Really an Option?...*22*

What's in a Word? 23

The Natural Choice..24

3   Weighing the Risks and Rewards   25

The Birth You Want..26

    Can You Really Do This?...*26*

    Can You Make the Commitment?...*27*

    What's in It for You?..*29*

History's Legacy 30

    The Invisible Threat of Infection *30*

    Crooked Bodies, Fragmented Design.......................................*31*

How Safe, Really, Is Natural Birth Today?.................................32
   Your Health Foundation *32*
   Multiples *33*
   What If You've Previously Had a C-Section? *33*
   When Loved Ones Don't Support Your Choices *34*
And the Winner Is ... Your Baby!..34
Feeling Confident About Your Decision....................................35

Part 2:   The Truth About Natural Childbirth   37

4   How Much Will It Hurt ... *Really?*   39
Cultural Origins of Painful Birth 40
Worries and Fears 41
So What *Do* You Feel During Labor?.......................................41
   Your Insensitive Cervix...*43*
   The Myth of the "Pain-Free" Surgical Birth.......................*44*
Those Wonderful Birth Hormones 44
   Oxytocin: Can You Feel the Love? *44*
   Endorphins: What a Rush! *45*
   Adrenaline: Hey, Baby ... Let's Go! *46*
The Power of Expectation 47
   Think Positively—It's No Cliché *47*
   This, Too, Shall Pass *48*
Methods to Maintain Your Comfort.......................................48
Orgasmic Birth...50
What Does Birth Feel Like to Your Baby?...............................51

5   Is Your Body in Shape for a Natural Birth?   53
Your Natural Body Is in Perfect Shape!...................................54
   Your Body Knows What Shape to Be In.................................*54*
   Stay Active!...*54*
   Water Workout *57*
   It's All in the Way You Carry Yourself................................*57*
The Matter of Weight...58
Eat Well, Eat Often 59
How's Your Health? 60
   Health Conditions...*60*
   Health Risks *61*

6 Is a Natural Birth Dangerous?   **63**

Everybody Worries 64

Birth's Mythology of Danger...64

When the Numbers Do the Talking 65

Birth Is Safe ... It's Intervention That's the Danger *66*

The "Do Something!" Syndrome *67*

Genuine Danger or Scare Tactic? 69

The Importance of Knowing Normal 70

Pressure's Rising *70*

The Incredible Placenta *71*

Focus on What Matters 73

7 Making a Choice: Midwife or Doctor?   **75**

Shop Around.. 76

Getting Down to Your Short List *77*

Go Together..*77*

Who's Who ... The Major Players 78

Midwives..79

Certified Nurse Midwife (CNM)...*80*

Direct-Entry Midwife *81*

Lay Midwife *82*

Doulas..82

Physicians 83

Surgical Specialist: The Obstetrician *84*

Emphasis on the Bigger Picture: The Family Practitioner............ *85*

Twenty Questions: Interviewing Your Provider-to-Be 86

Interview Questions for Your Provider-to-Be *87*

Making Sense of the Answers...*90*

8 Homebirth, Birthing Center, or Hospital?   **93**

The Right Place..94

Home Is Where the Heart Lives..94

Factors to Consider with a Homebirth....................................*96*

What About the Kids? *97*

Homebirth: The Politics and the Controversy............................*97*

Birthing Centers..98

The Midwifery Birthing Center..*99*

Hospital-Based Birthing Centers *100*

Ready for Anything: Hospital Birth...................................... 101
The Business of Birthing... 102
Safeguarding Your Options for Natural Birth in a Hospital 103
Shifting the Energy 104
A Not-So-Minor Detail: Who Pays? 104
Deciding What Works for You 105

Part 3:   Planning for a Natural Childbirth   107

9   What to Eat   109
Eating for You, Not Two 110
*Why Calories Count ... and Why You Shouldn't
  Count Calories*... 110
Focus on Nutrition, Not Weight....................................... 111
Big Babies.. 112
The Brewer Diet 113
Beef (or Bean) Up the Protein 114
Keep It Real... 116
Drink Up!.. 116
Eating During Labor 117

10   Yoga, Stretching, and Massage   119
Relaxin' with Relaxin 120
Yoga: As One 121
The Breath 122
Basic (Easy) Breathing.. 123
Complete (Three-Part) Breathing...................................... 123
Alternate Nostril Breathing.. 124
Poses... 125
Yoga in Labor and Birthing.. 127
Stretches: Range of Motion 128
Stretching Routine 128
Let the Water Carry You Away 129
Stretching During Labor and Birthing................................ 130
Massage: Hands On 131
Ah, That Feels Good!.. 131
Self-Massage... 132
Perineal Massage 132
Massage During Labor and Birthing................................... 133

11 Preparing for a Mindful Birth   **135**

Thought Bubbles: An Exercise in Mindfulness 136
Life Lives in the Moment 137
What If … 137
Fear, Stress, and Cortisol 138
Mind over Matter 139
    Share the Moment 140
    Beyond Birth 140
Below the Surface of Consciousness: Calming the Energy 141
    On Point: Acupressure 142
    Delving Deeper: Energy Methods 144
Stay Tuned 144

12 Support for Going Natural   **147**

Now Playing: Your Birth! 148
The Home Team 148
    Your Assignment Is … 149
    Final Preparations 150
Natural Birth in a Hospital 150
    Claim Your Space 151
    Dealing with Protocols and Routines 152
    Do a Doula 153
Support in a Birthing Center 154
Leave the Kitchen Sink; Bring Everything Else 154
All in the Family 155
    When Loved Ones Disagree 156
    Asking for Support and Understanding 157
Nearly a Year to Practice 157

Part 4: Natural Birthing Methods   **159**

13 Childbirth Preparation   **161**

Childbirth Education 161
    Core Essentials 162
    Who's Teaching? 163
    Free at Your Local Hospital! 164
Approaches That Support Natural Birth 165
    Birth Is Normal: The Lamaze Method 165
    Partners in Birthing: The Bradley Method 166
    HypnoBirthing: The Mongan Method 167

Preparation for Homebirth... 168
Finding the Classes That Are Right for You 168
Not for Birthing Women Only! 169

14 Waterbirth   171
Laboring Woman Defies Gravity! 172
The Many Benefits of Water in Labor and Birthing 173
Wait a Minute … Everything Has Stopped! 173
Birthing into Water... 174
Who Should Avoid Waterbirth?.. 175
Not Too Hot, Not Too Cold 176
Birthing Tub Considerations... 176
MacGyver Your Own Faucet Extension 177
Will a Regular Bathtub Do?.. 178
Running Water 179
Birthing Tubs and Hospitals... 179

15 Birth with Hypnosis   181
An Altered State of Attention 182
A Brief Hypnotic History... 183
What an Entrancing Experience!.. 183
How Hypnosis Works 184
Believing Is Being... 185
Practice Makes Permanent.. 185
Control Issues 186
Finding a Birth Hypnosis Program.. 186
Instructor Qualifications... 187
Partner Participation.. 188
Is It Real? 188
Surround Yourself with What You Want,
  Not What You Fear 189

16 Calling All Doulas   191
An Ancient Tradition 192
The Modern Doula 193
What Does a Doula Do?... 194
Birth Doula.. 195
Postpartum Doula 196
Does Your Baby Need a Doula, Too? 196
Doula Qualifications 197

Hiring a Doula 197

An Independent Doula 199

A Staff Doula 199

Collaborating for Your Best Birth 200

17 Making Your Birthing Preferences   **201**

What You Prefer 202

Put It in Writing 202

Say What You Want Your Birth Experience to Be 204

Make Your Preferences as Long as You Need Them to Be 206

Who Gets a Copy? 206

Deal Breakers 207

Can You Change Your Mind? 208

Stay Flexible 209

Expect the Best! 209

Part 5: Your Baby's Birthday Arrives!   **211**

18 Natural Labor   **213**

All the World's a Stage 214

Dress Rehearsal: Prelabor 215

Early Labor 216

Unplugged 217

The Misperception of Breaking Water 217

This Chair's Too Hard, It's Cold in Here, and Doesn't Anybody Know How to Make a Decent Sandwich? 218

Put Up Your Feet, Take a Rest 219

Honey, It's Time! 220

Transition 220

Staying True to Your Best Birth 221

19 The Nonmedicated Birth   **223**

"I Can't Do This Any Longer!" 223

Tuning in to Your Inner Messages 225

The Essence of Time 225

"I'll Save That Until I Really Need It" 226

Hello, Baby! 227

Your Body Knows When to Push 227

Eject! 229

Steady Does It Best 229

Stage Three: Birthing the Placenta......................................230
The Bigness of Birth...231

20 What if the Pain Is Too Much ... and Other Things That Can Happen 235

More Than You Bargained For 236
    A Crunch Start..237
    Too Much, Too Long..237
The Medication Decision 238
    Narcotic Medications..239
    The Epidural..240
    Laboring Down with an Epidural....................................242
Failure to Progress 243
My, What a Big Baby You Have 243
Bottom's Down 244
Oops, I Pooped 245
When It Comes to C-Section 246
Take a "Pass" on the Guilt Trip...247

Part 6: Welcoming Your New Baby **249**

21 Your Baby's First Moments, Naturally **251**

What an Amazing Thing You've Done! 252
    Onto Your Chest..252
    First Breath...253
    Unclamped and Uncut...254
    You Smell So Good!...255
The Sea Change of Your Baby's First 12 Hours......................255
    The Body Dynamic...256
    Testing, Testing..257
    More Endorphins..258
Talk to Your Baby 259

22 Postpartum: What You'll Feel Like **261**

Welcome to the Twilight Zone 262
    Another Hormonal Shift...262
    Feed Me! 263
    I Love My Baby ... May I Have Another Tissue, Please?........263
    A Little Help, Please..264
    Everybody Loves a Baby..265
Pace Yourself 266

Two Weeks: A Milestone 266
Baby Blues ... or Postpartum Depression? 266
   Causes and Treatments 268
   Compounding Factors 268
The Return of Real Life (SEX) 269
Your Path Is Unique.. 271

23 Breastfeeding, of Course   **273**

It's Not That Complicated ... Really! 274
   Belly to Belly: Helping Your Baby Latch 274
   Patience and Relaxation are Key 275
   Should You "Toughen" Your Nipples? 276
   Stick With It 277
When You Can't Breastfeed 278
Your Milk: The Perfect Baby Formula 278
   The Real Deal 279
   Is Your Baby Getting Enough? 279
   Poop 280
A Lifelong Foundation 281

24 You'd Do It All Again   **283**

With Woman 284
   The Secret 284
   Trust Yourself 285
   Catching Babies 286
Birth, the Greatest Story Ever Written 286
From the Waterfall to the Lighthouse............................ 287
Full Circle.. 289
Once More, with Gusto 289

Appendixes

  A Resources   **291**

  B Glossary   **297**

    Index   **301**

Foreword

Part of my job as a family doctor is to help women through their pregnancies and births. But I am first a woman and mother, and only then a doctor.

I have always loved being at a birth. I remember the first birth I witnessed as a medical student. It was a teenaged couple and they kissed the entire time. The oxytocin was flowing and the baby birthed easily. I felt like we were all intruding on something very sacred, very precious, and very private. Not many births throughout my career have been so passionate and easy. I have also seen how things can "go bad." I see how women too often aren't interested in taking the power to birth their own babies. I have seen how occasionally it really is so important to have doctors and surgeons around. But only occasionally.

Over the last twelve years of being around the medical field and birth (both as a medical student, a resident, and now as a family doctor), I have thought about the human birth puzzle a lot! Are we willing to give away the power of our births to prevent any possible danger from this natural process? Are we really willing to turn over one set of risks for another? Are we willing simply to give up the responsibility and the accomplishment to someone else? I hope not.

I believe strongly in prenatal care and having a trained birth attendant at every birth—be it a traditional birth attendant (TBA), a midwife, or a doctor. I believe in cesarean when it is truly needed. I believe in certain situations women require medical expertise. When people are sick, they need a doctor.

I don't believe in the vast majority of low-risk healthy women being afraid of the amazing things their bodies can do and therefore opting to have someone else "get the baby out." Too many doctors are too willing to take that responsibility from women when it isn't medically needed. It sets up a dangerous situation. If you help people who don't really need help, they are bound to blame you if things don't go well.

Being present and empowering women through birth is different than directing the process. You can even actively manage certain aspects of birth without intervening unnecessarily. People, and providers, don't feel like they are "doing anything" unless they are physically in motion. But giving high vibration and complete attention, and being a witness, can often be the only support a laboring woman needs.

And that brings me to my own birth. I knew I wanted a natural birth—defined for me as no hospital, no pain medication, and as little medical help as possible. I chose a certified nurse midwife (CNM) who had a birth center outside of Philadelphia, Barbara Di'Mato. She did birth center births and homebirths. She seemed like a smart cookie and I liked her midwifery partner, too. I enjoyed my prenatal visits with her where I weighed myself and dipped my own urine. I felt in charge of my pregnancy and supported. I was still low risk at the end of my prenatal care, and we agreed I was a good candidate for a homebirth. She started to prepare me mentally for how I might handle the pain of my birth process at home. I decided on Hypnobirthing.

It was a Thursday and I was supposed to take Advanced Cardiac Life Support (ACLS) in downtown Philadelphia the day I felt my waters start to leak out. I cancelled. I started to contract that night and by Friday I was in active labor. I was in and out of the bathtub—I wasn't interested in a full waterbirth but the warm water was so helpful during my strong contractions. My neighbor Michelle had birthed two babies at home herself and she acted as my doula. She had also helped a couple other friends at their births—truly an experienced birth support person! Her hands felt like healing salve on my body. Her touch was magical. I remember eating popsicles and talking with friends all day between contractions. I had a lot of people at my birth—some that had planned to come and some that just happened to call, heard I was in labor, so packed up a bag and started driving. I had nine women friends and my husband all there in my home supporting my birth.

By Saturday evening I was 8 centimeters, so my midwife and her nurse came to my home. After my midwife had spent several hours with me and I had not changed my cervix, she offered to break my forebag. I agreed and after that I felt the baby's head come down hard on my pelvic bones. I had a vision of opening a giant door to let a being from another world slip into reality. I needed to push! It felt so incredible to push! I pushed for what seemed like a long time. It felt somewhere between having to have a giant poop and an orgasm—not a bad feeling at all.

Then my baby was crowning and I felt some pain that was sharp and then my Leili slipped out and I grabbed her up onto my naked belly. She looked like a wilted purple iris and then she cried a little and opened her eyes. She became bubble-gum pink and she was quiet and thoughtful looking. I knew she was okay and I thought, "Oh my God, look what I've done!" I felt like a superhero. I felt the power of the universe move through me and there was complete stillness and everyone was speaking but their words had deeper meaning than what they were saying. The gathering of all the souls at my daughter's birth made me weep.

I stayed in a blissful state for many days and weeks. It was one of the most amazing experiences in my life—certainly *the* most amazing until that point. I grew up in that moment and I realized I was ready to be a mother—to take the role of mother to my baby and the role of "mother" in society. This birth … it was important to me and I did it. I had many helpers but at the moment that most mattered, only I could do the work.

I may not have the birth story that calls to your heart—but that is why you must create your own! I may not agree with every aspect of this book as a doctor or as a woman—but I do agree with the idea that each woman needs to find her own way, her own story. Women should have choices about how they birth their babies, and I feel strongly that a natural birth can be a mystical and life-changing experience for many.

I don't ever want to take power away from the women I help to birth their babies. I believe there are many good providers who feel the same—both midwives and doctors. I also think that when women in society are not oppressed and disempowered they will birth better and a more enlightened planet will be had by all! So if you intend to have a natural birth, let all your fears go, do whatever it takes, and most of all believe that it can happen.

—Jennifer Phillips, M.D., May 2009

Introduction

How wonderful ... you're having a baby! Maybe this is your first birth, and you want to experience the fullness of birthing—the bringing of new life into the world. It is one of the most powerful and empowering experiences a woman can have. Birth is also the most natural and amazing of experiences, and your body is uniquely suited for and perfectly capable of it.

You have so many more choices than what to pack in your overnight bag for that clichéd mad dash to the hospital! There need not—and should not, for most women— even *be* a mad dash to *anywhere*. When you tune in to your body and the changes that take place to accommodate the new life growing within you, you realize that you really are designed to do this—and you don't need someone else telling you how to breathe and when to push. Exploring the full range of all your birthing options can only make you more confident as you look forward to the happy day when you welcome your baby into your arms—and being confident is the key to having your best possible birth. There's everything to celebrate and nothing to fear about birth, yet many myths and misunderstandings shroud the process of birth. In writing this book, it's our desire to cut through the misinformation and present the facts so you feel confident and strong in your ability to have a natural birth and to be fully aware and participate in the intensity of your body's ultimate effort.

Expert author Jenny West brings extensive experience as a midwife and delightful, down-to-earth humor when explaining and describing all the changes your body undergoes as it prepares for the momentous adventure of birthing. By the time you've finished reading this book, you'll feel as if she's your midwife! You'll also feel centered in yourself about the birthing experience you want for you and your baby and knowledgeable about how to make that happen.

Happy reading, and happy birthing!

How to Use This Book

We've organized this book into six parts that follow your progression through pregnancy and planning for your birth experience.

Part 1, "You're Having a Baby, Naturally!", explores the concepts and approaches toward birth throughout history and in current times. These chapters take a look at beliefs, misinformation, and weighing the balance of what's best for you and the birth experience you desire.

Part 2, "The Truth About Natural Childbirth," delves into the heart of the issues and controversies surrounding medicated versus nonmedicated birth. These chapters investigate and discuss what it means to have a natural birth; the different kinds of practitioners who assist with birthing and how to choose the one who's right for you; and whether you want to birth your baby at home, in a birthing center, or in a hospital.

Part 3, "Planning for a Natural Childbirth," gets down to the details of preparing your body and mind for a natural birth. You're eating for two now, but not in the way you might think. Is your body ready for this great effort? These chapters discuss nutrition, exercise, and activity and mindful approaches to help you become ready for birthing and to give your baby the best possible start.

Part 4, "Natural Birthing Methods," explores the many ways to work with your body's natural efforts and mechanisms for keeping you calm, relaxed, and comfortable during labor and birthing. These chapters look at Lamaze breathing, the Bradley Method, waterbirth, hypnosis, and other approaches. The more you know, the better you'll be able to manage whatever circumstances arise.

Part 5, "Your Baby's Birthday Arrives!", celebrates your baby's journey from your womb to your arms. Chapters explain exactly what happens during labor, from the hormones and other natural substances your body produces to ready your body for birthing to contractions and the changes that take place to allow your baby to leave your body. What happens when things don't go quite according to plan, however? We cover that, too!

Part 6, "Welcoming Your New Baby," looks at the first minutes, days, and weeks that follow your baby's birth. Chapters discuss the postpartum hormone rollercoaster, your emotions, breastfeeding, and of course the joys of getting to know this new person.

Extras

There's so much to share with you about the magnificent journey of natural birth! Sometimes we have something to tell you that's a side step from our discussion or important enough for special attention. When this happens, you'll see one of these special boxes:

 Oh, Baby!

These boxes alert you to concerns, issues, and potential risks or cautions.

 Trusty Midwife Tips

These boxes give practical tidbits, advice, and suggestions.

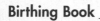

Birthing Book

These boxes define terms that may be unfamiliar to you or that have a specific meaning in this book.

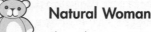

Natural Woman

These boxes contain anecdotes, brief personal experiences, and quotes about natural birth.

Acknowledgments

Just as it takes a village to raise a child, it takes a community to write a book such as this—and we wish to acknowledge those who created the opportunity. We extend our appreciation and gratitude to the women and their partners who shared their birthing stories and experiences for this book; to Lee Ann Chearney, creative director of Amaranth IlluminAre, without whom there would be a very different and boringly ordinary book on the shelf; and to our dedicated editorial team at Alpha Books.

Jenny gives special thanks to every birthing woman, family, and student of birth and baby, for they have created the ever-changing, ever-expanding body of knowledge to allow her the honor of continuing to attend births. Says Jenny, "I am constantly amazed at how much mothers and babies have to teach us." And finally, Jenny honors the guidance of intuition, instinct, and mentors who help keep all the participants in a birth listening to what they already know and support them to be courageous enough to do it.

Special Thanks to the Technical Reviewer

The Complete Idiot's Guide to Natural Childbirth was reviewed by a physician expert who double-checked the accuracy of what you'll learn here to help us ensure that this book gives you everything you need to know about natural childbirth. We extend our thanks to Jennifer Phillips, M.D., and especially thank her and her daughter Leili for sharing, in the foreword, their own wonderful natural birth story with us and with our readers.

Dr. Phillips is an assistant professor at the University of New Mexico Department of Family and Community Medicine. Her special interests are women's health and reproduction, obstetrics, pediatrics, and preventative care. She comes from a long line of educators and is excited about the opportunity to empower those who would like to learn about medicine. Dr. Phillips practices patient-centered medicine, and she seeks to inspire her patients to be attentive to living healthy lives, involving the body, mind, and spirit. Dr. Phillips is a native New Mexican and she enjoys being in the mountains and the city with her little girl Leili; they like to hike, paint, and dance together.

Trademarks

All terms mentioned in this book that are known to be or are suspected of being trademarks or service marks have been appropriately capitalized. Alpha Books and Penguin Group (USA) Inc. cannot attest to the accuracy of this information. Use of a term in this book should not be regarded as affecting the validity of any trademark or service mark.

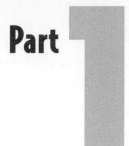

Part 1

You're Having a Baby, Naturally!

What could be more natural than birth? Yet, throughout history, misinformation and misunderstanding have shrouded this amazing journey. Today's women (and their partners) are reclaiming their right to experience birth fully informed, alert, and participatory. Whatever natural birth means for you, you can have it! The chapters in Part 1 explore the history of birth, take a look at how it came to be that birth is considered a medical condition, discuss the startling rate of medical interventions including cesarean sections, and explore what it means to plan for a natural birth.

Celebrating Your Pregnancy

In This Chapter

- ◆ Oh, the stories we hear!
- ◆ Create the birth story you want to experience—and tell
- ◆ Dispelling the myths of birth
- ◆ Taking back birth: your body knows how to do this!

When you decide on a natural birth, you embark on a journey of personal exploration, of loving your body and your whole self, of trusting your inner wisdom, and of bonding with the new life growing within you. On your baby's birthday, you'll be ready for the profound transformation of the birth experience in all its amazing power, confidence, and beauty. Nearly every woman who's had a natural birth views the experience as empowering and life-altering. She creates a new sense of self and a new measure for all she does from now on. She knows without any doubt that she can trust herself, fully and completely.

It sounds somewhat cliché to say that natural birth is the ultimate empowerment, but it is unbelievably empowering to take yourself well beyond what are considered the normal or daily limits of body and mind, well beyond what you thought was possible. If you've got more questions than answers, that's fine—and natural. But take heart—all that you need for this journey is already within you!

The Birth Story

As you prepare for birth, you'll have lots of information—some accurate, some not—to sift through. Your baby is counting on you to figure out what you both need so that you can have the best possible birth. Birth is a joyous event, and you should be able to anticipate it with calm confidence and delight. What have you heard, or experienced yourself, about birth? How many times have you heard the story, and how does the story change with each retelling? What's the first birth story you ever heard? Take a few minutes right now to write it down, in as much detail as you can remember:

_____

_____

_____

_____

_____

_____

Who first told you this story, and how did it come up? How old were you? Do you remember how you felt when you first heard it? When you read this story out loud now, how does it make you feel about birth? What kinds of things are women saying to you now that you're pregnant? Does birth sound like an experience of joy, or is it simply something you have to go through to hold your baby in your arms?

Natural Woman _____

Do you know the story of your own birth? Where and how were you born? Even if you've heard it before, it's often interesting to have your mother tell you your birth story now. If possible, ask your mother some of the questions that you're contemplating now about the birth of your baby. If there are others who can tell their versions of the story of your birth, this will add richness and new perspective. The result could connect you to your own place along the spectrum of motherhood in some unique and unexpected ways.

What if this were the kind of birth story women told each other:

I watched my birth video a few days after the birth, and I could see how calm and focused I looked, even though my thoughts were all jumbled in my mind during that part of my labor. I felt like the labor was long, and there was a point in the labor where it didn't seem I was making much progress—that nothing was really happening—especially for all the effort my body was making. When I got in the birthing tub and I did some focused breathing and grunting, I felt better and decided that all I could do is relax and let my body take over. I found out after the birth that I was in the tub for about an hour, but at the time I really had no idea how long it was. Then, I had a big urge to push, and the baby's head and shoulders came out all at once. I put my hands down to take my baby as she was born. My baby was born into my own arms. I couldn't believe it when Jenny told me my beautiful daughter weighed almost 10 pounds! I felt fine the next day, like giving birth had been nothing out of the ordinary—although it was, of course, a most extraordinary experience that I'll always remember and cherish.

Imagine what it would be like if every time women talked to each other about their births, they felt happy and pleased with their experiences! This is how most women *should* be talking about their births, not as if birth is a contest about who had the worst suffering or the longest labor. The day your baby comes into your arms should be something you relish and can't wait for—not something you fear and doubt.

I Had a Great Birth, and Everyone Hates Me!

We're not exactly encultured to believe that birth is a joyful experience. It's good in its outcome, yes (and in its conception, too!). But birthing as joyful in itself … well, that's harder to believe for a lot of women. We're more likely to hear stories of pain and difficulty. Who wants to sign on for *that?* Not you! That's not the birth experience you're seeking, to be sure—which is one reason why you're reading this book. Nor is it the birth experience any woman needs to have.

Maybe you've already had a birth experience that wasn't quite the birth story you want to tell, so you want to try something different this time around. Maybe you feel that if you learn more about all your different options, you'll be better able to shape this birth. No matter what birth stories you've heard or birth experiences you've had yourself, *this* birth will be unique. Its story is yet to be written.

Inside the Birth Myths

Myths about childbirth are so much a part of the fabric of our beliefs that we have a hard time setting them aside—even when we know or suspect they're either not true or there's a lot more to them than meets the ear. Let's take a look at some of the common myths about birth.

Myth No. 1: Birth has to be an ordeal of pain and misery.

Reality: Birth is one of the most profound and intense physical and emotional experiences you can have. Your body produces hundreds of hormones and other biochemicals to move that baby from your belly to your arms. When you know exactly what is happening, you can focus on allowing your body to do what it needs—and already knows how—to do. Does birth hurt? Most women will say "Yes." But your perception and experience of that pain changes vastly when you understand that it has benefit and ends when that purpose is fulfilled. You learn methods to go with the flow of and actively assist, rather than fight, your body's work.

Myth No. 2: You have to go to the hospital to have a baby.

Reality: In the United States, about 98 percent of births do take place in hospitals or hospital-affiliated birthing centers, so it's little wonder this is our expectation! (In Holland, as sophisticated a society as any in our modern world, by contrast, more than half of births take place at home with midwives in attendance—though the government in Holland mandates the number of women who homebirth with a midwife through government policy.) In reality, only about 10 percent of birthing women need what doctors and hospitals have to offer. However, hospital birthing is so deeply ingrained in our culture that often it never occurs to us that we might want, and can have, something different—or that something different might actually be better for us.

> **Trusty Midwife Tips**
>
> Even if you decide you prefer to birth your baby in a hospital, look around at different hospitals if this is an option where you live. Although to a certain degree a hospital is a hospital, protocols, policies, and practices vary widely even within the same community.

Myth No. 3: Labor has to be long.

Reality: Labor is as long as your baby needs it to be. What matters most is your ability to work with your labor to let your baby's transition from the womb to the world occur as naturally and gently as possible. Labor is work (that's why we call it *labor!*). It takes a type of focus that you'll never experience in any other context and maybe have never experienced before. But it's work that your body and your baby know how to do and have been preparing to do.

The challenge is in being willing to let that work unfold. Once labor is underway, interruptions and interventions break your concentration and focus. Many interruptions are well-intended, such as asking if you'd like another blanket or adjusting your pillow because it looks uncomfortable. Some interruptions are driven by protocols, such as taking your vital signs or fetal monitoring on a certain schedule. Such interruptions can, and usually do, change the rhythm of your labor—sometimes causing the natural flow of your body's efforts to slow or even stop.

Interventions are intended to change the flow of your body's efforts, usually to "get things moving." Common interventions include drugs to stimulate contractions, and "breaking the waters" (rupturing the membranes surrounding the baby). However, counter to their intent, interventions can create the very situations that can cause your labor to be longer and more painful! And unfortunately, pain relief medications (including epidural) further slow the processes of labor. Yet, interruptions and interventions are so commonplace in current birthing that we don't even consider them as factors that can make labor longer.

Myth No. 4: Once you decide to take the path of a natural birth at home, you have to stay at home no matter what.

Reality: Why would you *have* to stay at home? Are there guards at the door? Nope! Homebirth is among the choices you can make for the birth experience you want to have. But there's no in-or-out rule. You can change your mind and go to a hospital or a birthing center if you want. Or, circumstances may change such that you need medical care—making the hospital the place for the birth. Birth is, after all, dynamic and ever-changing.

Trusty Midwife Tips

Although birth is a universal process—the same across cultures and throughout history—it's nonetheless a unique and personal experience for each woman. Every mother's body does the same things to birth a baby. What we can influence through conscious effort, however, is how long it takes, what the baby feels, and what the mother feels during the process. Only you can make the choices and decisions that are right for you, your baby, and your birth experience.

Myth No. 5: You can't have pain medications at home.

Reality: Well, you certainly can't have an epidural at home! (See Chapter 4 about how an epidural affects you, your baby, and the birth.) However, there are many other methods for increasing relaxation, improving your comfort, and trusting your birth process that don't involve drugs. The focus should be on relaxation and confidence that you are doing what feels best to you—not necessarily on medications that completely alter the birthing process and often your awareness of it, may create doubt in you about your ability to birth your baby, and often make you later regret saying okay to offered intervention.

Write Your Own Birth Story

Now it's time for you to write your own birth story—a story of your baby's birth that you want to tell over and over to anyone who'll listen.

Sure, you could choose to sit back and go along for the ride. After all, your baby's going to be born whether or not you participate in a conscious, intentional way. There's nothing wrong with making such a choice, and you might come to it as the best option for you after you've explored all the possibilities. But we're pretty sure you're reading this book because you want to do more than lounge in the passenger's seat!

Your baby is counting on you to pick the best foods, environments, care providers, support, education, and friends to share in this amazing experience. Your baby trusts you to choose the best way and place to have the birth and to take charge of anything else that affects this time in your life. As you read further in this book, you'll see how all of your choices, both small and large, add up. One decision sets in motion another decision … and another, and another ….

You might be having your first, second, or eighth baby. But each baby gets only *one* birth. There's no "do-over." Only you can decide how this birth is going to be.

Reclaiming Birth

Growing numbers of women are reclaiming birth as the natural, incredible experience that it is. We're not as connected anymore, in our modern culture, to women's wisdom. All of that changes the moment you find out you're pregnant, because you're now carrying another life within you. Every woman who has birthed before you now stands beside you, allowing you to access your inner wisdom. But the core of it really is this: trusting your own instincts and intuition. No one can care more about you, your baby, and your birth than you do.

When the time comes for your baby's birthday, no one knows better than *you* what's normal—what is needed and wanted and what isn't. You're intimately familiar with every subtlety of your baby's movements and personality and with every subtlety of your own body through the course of your pregnancy. Why would you want to check all this at the door just because it's your baby's birthday? You are the expert on this little being. Trust that, especially when other people may be telling you something different. No matter where you are in your pregnancy, when you realize something may not be working for you, you can take steps to change course to ensure your best birth.

Natural Woman

"We must relearn to trust the feminine, to trust women and their bodies as authoritative regarding the children they carry and the way they must birth them. When women and their families make their own decisions during pregnancy, when they realize their own wisdom regarding birth and its place in their lives, they have a foundation of confidence and sensitivity that will not desert them as parents."

—Elizabeth Davis, American midwife, educator, and women's health specialist

Giving Yourself the Best Preparation

You wouldn't run the Honolulu Marathon after reading the event brochure just because you've never been to Hawaii and what's a little bit of running, anyway? Why, only last week you chased the dog halfway across the park. The human body, after all, does have the natural ability to run. But it's highly unlikely you'd make it to even the first checkpoint. If you really wanted to run the Honolulu Marathon, you'd stick the brochure on the fridge and then devour all the information—from nutrition and hydration to stretches and running techniques—that you could get your hands on.

You'd subscribe to magazines, scour websites and blogs, and talk to people who've run marathons. You'd check out maps of the race route and investigate the weather history. You'd sign on with a trainer or running group and begin months in advance to prepare your body and your mind. You'd give it your absolute all, knowing that when you bring everything into focus for those five or six hours of intensive effort there'll be no words to describe your ecstasy at crossing that finish line!

Oh, Baby!

When you do your online research, be sure to look for reputable sources. Some information posted online is not quite true or is flat-out wrong. We include a good list of online resources in the resource appendix at the back of this book.

It's much the same for a natural birth. Your body has the design and ability to do it, just like with running. But is it in shape and conditioned for such a monumental effort as a natural birth? Are you ready in your thoughts and emotions? Natural birth, like a marathon, is no dog chase through the park. You'll need to study and practice, starting now, to get your body and mind in shape. Does it take time and effort? Surely, it does. But you've got this book as a great foundation for your preparation.

Everything You Need Is Already Within You

There are no great secrets when it comes to natural birth. Having a natural birth is more about unlearning fears and worries than about learning methods and techniques. All those many millennia ago, when women birthed as though birth were simply another activity in the day, there was no one standing around saying, "Wow, that's gotta hurt!"

Birthing was simply something women did. They breathed, grunted, groaned, moved around, and got into whatever positions their bodies wanted to take. Your body already knows what to do and how to do it, and although birthing classes will teach you many positions to take, the main thing to learn is to let your body guide you.

That said, it's important, too, to have people with you at the time of your birthing who support your decisions about the birth experience you desire and who can encourage you in ways that will help you achieve that experience. Even such seemingly simple things as having someone to get you a drink or something to eat, to rub your back, or to just sit there with you can give you the boost you need to reach a little bit deeper into your inner resources to regain confidence and trust that you *do* know how to do this.

You Have More Choices Than You Think

It's true that birth is inevitable. If you do absolutely nothing to prepare for birth, your baby will still come out of your body when it's time. So why go through the process of making choices and decisions beforehand? Why not wait until you have to address them? You could do that, of course. Maybe you won't even have to deal with some of the questions that right now perplex you. But the problem with this approach is that not making a choice is itself a choice. We call it decision by default, and it puts other people in charge of all sorts of things from whether you can eat a turkey sandwich during labor because you're hungry and that's what sounds good to you, to whether the lights are bright or dim, to if you get an epidural.

Every woman wants to know, moments, months, and even years after her birth, that she made the right decisions for herself and for her baby. Yet it might feel like many decisions aren't truly yours to make. After all, no one knows what might happen during birth. You could put months of time and effort into preparation, only to find yourself in circumstances beyond your control that dictate the path of your birthing experience. While this is certainly true, very few situations have *no* options. So the more you know, the better able you are to participate in choosing the ones that are most closely aligned with the birth experience you desire—and that are best for you and your baby.

Pregnancy is a continuum of choices and decisions, from picking the baby's name to choosing what color to paint the baby's room to what car seat and baby furniture to get. Most women have little trouble with these kinds of details; they're tangible and well within control, even when you and your partner or others disagree about them. When it comes to the long-awaited conclusion to pregnancy, the joyous moment of birth, many women suddenly feel that events determine choices and decisions, and that other people know better than they do what's right and best. In reality, though, it's often the other way around: choices and decisions determine events. And nearly always, *you* are the one who knows best what's happening with your body, in your birthing, and for yourself and your baby.

> **Trusty Midwife Tips**
>
> Sometimes the realization that there are so many options when it comes to birthing is overwhelming, and you begin to get caught up in worrying about making the right choices even before you make very many choices at all. If you feel this happening, just take a few calming breaths, close your eyes, and invite your baby to show you her birth.

Take the Lead!

Women are so strong and capable, yet somehow we've come to view birth less as a natural experience and more as a medical event—a perspective that has its roots in the right place but that has grown well beyond its original motivation. It's not easy to undo entrenched beliefs and practices, even when the evidence fails to support them. It's such an automatic assumption that doctors deliver babies in hospitals. Indeed, the first suspicion of pregnancy commonly leads (after those five home pregnancy tests that you do yourself) straight to the doctor's office.

From this pregnant moment on, you have a say in how you feel and what you do *every day. You* determine what you eat, how much you sleep, and how much physical activity you get. These are key factors that shape your pregnancy and your potential birth experiences. Is your baby's journey toward birth an experience to explore and savor or is it a destination-driven, "Are we there yet?" drudge? A journey is so much more exciting and satisfying when you participate in getting to the destination!

You can prepare yourself—body, mind, and spirit—to nurture the new life growing within you and ready yourself to bring this baby into the world. It matters what you do each day, how you feel about labor and birth, what you listen to, what you watch on TV, and who you invite to participate in this amazing time. What a joy and honor for you to be fully present, aware, and participating in this amazing experience of giving birth!

The Least You Need to Know

- The stories you hear from other women, true or not, shape your perceptions and expectations about pregnancy and birth; you can choose the ones you want to hear.

- Your body and your baby are designed to give birth, and they know how to do this; it's a shared effort.

- You have choices … lots of choices!

- Listen to your instincts; they'll guide you right and true.

What Does It Mean to Give Birth Naturally?

In This Chapter

- ◆ Birth by natural design
- ◆ Natural birth is more about *how*, not *where*, you birth
- ◆ The domino effect of intervention
- ◆ The power of language

On the surface, the definition of natural birth is pretty straightforward: it's birth without *unnecessary* interventions that alter the innate process of birthing. The midwife or doctor who attends a natural birth takes a low profile unless circumstances require otherwise, supporting and encouraging the woman, though allowing the birthing process to unfold in its own rhythm and time. The goal of everyone present is to help the birthing mother stay relaxed, focused, and confident. A partner, close friend, sister, mom, or even the new baby's siblings may be the ones who bring you hot tea, massage your back, and softly ooh and ahh when those little eyes take their first look at the outside world.

But there's no single definition, no encyclopedia or rulebook, for natural birth. Within the range of what it means to have a birth without interventions, natural birth means something different and unique to each woman who considers it. Some women define natural birth as absolutely no assistance of any kind from anyone, leaving everything in the hands of Mother Nature. And some women think natural birth means wearing no makeup! However, most women—and most natural births—are somewhere in between.

Who's in Charge? You!

Birth is the most natural process humans have. We wouldn't be a prolific, thriving species if birth were as complicated as it sometimes appears to be. We tend to lose sight of this fact, though, immersed as we are in a culture that equates birth with due dates, ultrasounds, and the quickest route to the hospital. We like facts, data, and action. Birth, by contrast, functions within a universe of its own creation. Establish whatever "due" date you like; the day will come when *your baby* is ready!

It may seem a little odd at first to contemplate a birth in which there's not someone else taking control and directing things, but instead there's *you* … fully knowledgeable, capable, and empowered to birth your baby. Choosing a natural birth does not mean you're turning away from approaches that could create a comfortable birth experience for you, although this is a common misperception. Rather, choosing a natural birth means you're climbing out of the passenger's seat to get behind the wheel. This is *your* journey, and you're taking charge. Why not take the scenic route, the route *you* want to take? You're going to travel this specific passage only once, no matter how many births you have.

Restoring birth to the context of a natural process shifts everything about it. In the course of your normal daily activities do you ask someone else if you can have a drink of water or eat a sandwich? Highly unlikely! Instead, you drink when you're thirsty and eat when you're hungry. Your body sends the signals and you respond. Why should it be any different when you're birthing? If you're feeling hungry, your body's telling you it needs more energy. Drinking keeps you hydrated, which supports everything your body needs to do as it prepares for your baby to leave its confines. However, elements such as these have not so much to do with *where* you birth (although that can play a role), as is a common belief, but rather with *how* you birth— and that you birth with intent and awareness.

It's About You, Too

Natural birth is, of course, about your baby. This is her birth, after all. But birth is also about you. You are the one who's in the world. Your baby's still waiting to join you. For all of the latest and greatest technology, there's as yet no way to open a window and peek inside your uterus to see what's going on in there during birth! Nearly always, what's good for you is what's good for your baby. When you're calm, comfortable, and relaxed, your baby is, too.

Often, an undue emphasis on trying to determine what's going on with the baby during birth leads to all kinds of interruptions and interventions that interfere with your efforts to birth your baby. All that checking and monitoring, poking and prodding, measuring and gauging may provide a whole lot of information, but to what end? Sometimes not the one you had in mind. Information for the sake of information may be interesting but it's not very helpful for you, your birth experience, or your baby.

But I'm Not Really the "Earth-Mother" Type

The entire natural birth idea invokes a sense of, well, primal earthiness that not all women may find appealing or comfortable. If you're one of those women, you can relax and keep reading. No one's going to make you put on a tie-dyed skirt and braid your hair. You are who you are, and you owe it to yourself and your baby to sculpt the kind of birth you want to have. You may be surprised at how "Mother-Earthy" concepts provide a tremendous amount of comfort and common sense.

Another common belief about natural birth is that it's a birth at home. It is for many women, but not for all. Natural birth is about *how*, far more than *where*, you have your baby. That said, it's much easier to have a natural birth at home than in a birthing center or hospital (most birthing centers in the United States are part of, or owned by, hospitals).

Some women choose to birth at home because home is where they're most comfortable. They may want to feel free to roam about in a skirt, in a favorite bathrobe, or in nothing at all! They may want people with them who can be present without being intrusive. They may want to fix their own snacks, move back and forth from the birthing tub to the outside garden as the mood moves them, and even read or nap if that's what they feel like doing. In other words, they want to be free to do what they want to do, when they want to do it, and how they want to do it—without time, protocols, liability, and other external factors defining their choices.

You may decide on a natural birth and choose to birth in a birthing center or a hospital—both are possible when you have a supportive provider (although hospitals present more of a challenge). Chapters 7 and 8 discuss the choosing of your provider and birth location. In Chapter 17, you'll find out how to write your birth story as you want to see it unfold. But it's never too early to start thinking about it and jot down some notes as you're reading, listening to what other women have to say about natural birth, and thinking about your options. The more time and attention you place on getting what you want, the closer you will be to having a birth you desire.

> **Trusty Midwife Tips** _____
>
> We can't overemphasize the importance of having a clear intention when it comes to your vision of your birthing experience. But at the same time, it's essential to be able to let go and remain fully in the moment—moment by moment—as the birth unfolds. This is the great paradox of birth!

What a Natural Birth Is *Not*

Sometimes it's enlightening to look at what natural birth is *not:* pain medications, routinely "breaking the waters" (*amniotomy*), drugs to induce or augment labor (such as Pitocin), epidurals, regional nerve blocks, *episiotomies*, vacuum extractors, IVs, electronic fetal monitoring, or c-sections. (More about interventions later in this chapter.) Natural birth also is not bright lights, loud voices, and a merry-go-round of personnel.

> **Birthing Book** _____
>
> An **amniotomy** is the artificial rupture of the amniotic membranes using a hook-like device inserted into the vagina. An **episiotomy** is a surgical incision to widen the vaginal opening.

Not that any of these actions is inherently bad; each has its place and many women benefit from their appropriate use. Even that ever-rotating parade of staff can provide much-needed fresh perspective, bringing new energy and new suggestions. Yet many of these interventions are now so routine in the hospital settings where most women have their babies that the experience of birth many times becomes traumatic. This is not how birth should be, no matter where you have your baby.

Most certainly, a healthy baby and a healthy mom are the most important goals in every birth, but you need specific reasons and precise benefits so you can make the decisions that are right for you and your baby. What is the intended outcome of the proposed intervention? What are the risks? What happens if you delay a bit longer? What happens if you say "no"? These are key answers you need to make informed choices.

Natural Woman

Some women get a little queasy or are put off with the idea that birth is messy and bloody. But most people have only ever seen birth portrayed in movies and on TV, which often exaggerates what actually happens so that you'll be sure to watch. There's no such thing as gallons of amniotic fluid or extreme pain being the sign of the first contraction. Often in the movies, the only difference between having a heart attack and having a baby is whether the actress grabs her chest or bends over and cradles her belly!

The Winding Road of Birth Intervention

How did we get so far away from natural birth that it's become an experience of special request (and often one of dedicated effort as well)? It's perhaps best to say simply that the road to intervention is paved with good intentions. The most significant, and enduring, of these interventions are pain relief and surgical birth.

Sleep Tight

Anesthetized birth debuted in the nineteenth century with the desire to help women have an easier time during childbirth. Doctors didn't really know all that much about pregnancy and birth—and they knew even less about how to use the body's own mechanisms to support labor and birth. And by this time, neither did most women because they went to doctors and to hospitals to have their babies. Mostly, what doctors knew about birth were its complications and pain. Pelvic deformities were especially problematic.

In 1845, American surgeon Crawford Long (1815–1878) used ether—which, at the time, had been known solely for the entertaining intoxication it produced as a party drug—to anesthetize a woman during a particularly grueling labor. Not only did the woman lose consciousness, but she also remembered nothing of the experience afterward. She and her doctor were amazed and happy, and the baby was fine. Scottish physician Sir James Simpson (1811–1870) used chloroform for the same purpose two years later, and soon every doctor carried these two chemicals in his black bag. We hesitate to call them anything kinder; in addition to knocking consciousness out of the picture, ether and chloroform are also strong solvents. Later, as with nearly everything that seems too good to be true, it became clear that these new anesthetics, as they became known, had significant risks for both mother and baby.

With advances in pharmacology in the early decades of the twentieth century, new drugs and combinations became available for surgery. These anesthetic methods quickly crossed over to birthing. From the 1930s to the 1960s, many women submitted to "twilight sleep" (an injected combination of the drugs morphine and scopolamine) as birth became imminent—and returned to groggy consciousness some hours later to find that they'd been sliced, extracted, and sutured and were without any memory whatsoever of the birth. Most were not permitted to hold their babies (who were groggy themselves), except for feeding, until they were permitted to go home. Mother and baby of course required close medical attention; both had been significantly traumatized and very drugged. Unfortunately, their shared helplessness further entrenched the belief that birth was a medical matter.

Birthing Book

An **epidural** is a form of regional anesthesia in which an anesthetic agent is injected into the space around the spinal cord in the lower back. The effect is to numb sensation (including voluntary movement) in the lower part of the body.

In the 1970s, anesthesia during birth took a turn with the increasing use of the *epidural*. Today, the epidural is ubiquitous; nearly two thirds of women who birth their babies in hospitals do so while awake and alert but numbed from belly to toes. A woman who receives an "epidural lite" (a smaller dose of anesthetic) may have enough sensation and control to feel when she needs to push. Most women lose the ability to feel what's happening in their bodies, however, requiring the doctor's assistance (and sometimes vacuum extraction or surgical birth) to get the baby out.

Natural Woman

A certified professional midwife (CPM), Ina May Gaskin (1940–) is credited with restoring midwifery and natural birth in the United States. In 1971, Ina May and her husband, Stephen, left San Francisco's famed Haight-Ashbury district for rural Tennessee where they founded the Farm, a still-thriving commune. Ina May developed a technique, now known as the Gaskin Maneuver, for helping a baby's shoulders rotate through the birth path for a normal, healthy, vaginal birth. She has attended more than 1,200 births and today teaches at the Farm Midwifery Center and lectures around the world to packed audiences.

But also in the 1970s came the first wave of women who decided *not* to go to the hospital to birth—women who were disgruntled with the manhandling of a woman's body during birth and with standard practices that took her baby away from her right after birth. The era of free love also brought in the concept among women that "My body is just fine!", and the premise of "back to nature" came to encompass lifestyle in a broad way. During this time, Ina May Gaskin—who would later become known as the "mother of midwifery"—cofounded the Farm, a commune that quickly became a mecca for natural, noninterventive birth.

What Did Caesar Have to Do with It?

Legend widely credits ancient Roman ruler Julius Caesar (100–44 B.C.E.) with the name associated with surgical birth: the *cesarean section*. The details of the association vary, but the general concept is that Julius Caesar or one of his ancestors was born by this method. Another story holds that Caesar (whether Julius or someone else) proclaimed that a baby was to be saved no matter what and instructed goat herders (qualified for the task because of their expertise in castrating goats) to slice the mother open to retrieve the baby. Talk about pressure to perform well in birth, knowing you'd be killed to save the baby—no wonder we have such subconscious fears about birth!

> **Birthing Book**
>
> A **cesarean section,** or c-section, is a surgical birth in which the surgeon makes an incision into the mother's abdomen and then into the uterus and removes the baby through the incision.

Like most legends, these stories fail to stand up to examination. We do know that from ancient times until about the 1950s, c-sections were desperate efforts to save an unborn baby after its mother died. (And we know Julius Caesar's mother lived to be 66, making it highly unlikely that Caesar's birth was, well, by c-section.) Another theory proposes a now-forgotten derivation arising from Latin terminology. No matter its origins, today we know surgical birth best as a c-section. You might see the full term spelled "caesarean" in countries other than the United States.

In the beginning, this major operation was intended as a last-ditch measure—never used casually or as an option. With the advent of antibiotics and predictable anesthesia after World War II—both lessons of combat—surgery of all kinds, including c-section, became commonplace. By the 1970s, c-section was a routine procedure (at least, from the hospital's perspective). By 2005, nearly one in three babies in the United States entered the world via surgical birth. Women who expect a c-section to relieve them from their fear of birth pain are in for a rude shock, however: most women need six weeks to recover from the operation, so walking, getting up to go to the bathroom, lifting a baby from the bed to the breast, rolling over, getting dressed, and just about every aspect of activity hurts and often requires lots of help from others.

The Regulation of Birth

Most countries today have laws and regulations regarding birthing, ostensibly to safe-guard women from charlatans and frauds who would do them harm. There is merit in the intent behind those efforts; we *do* want to know that the people helping us give birth have the knowledge, training, and skill to do so. But an unintended effect, damaging in other ways, is a deeper ingraining of not only the belief but the *expectation* that women are not capable of doing what their bodies are designed for them to do.

Birth has become a formalized practice of medicine with legal boundaries and requirements—some of which make natural birth as it existed before medical birth illegal. In some parts of the United States, Canada, and many countries in Europe, it's against the law for anyone other than an appropriately licensed practitioner to assist with a birth and for fathers to catch their own babies.

Same Goal, Divergent Paths

American poet Robert Frost (1874–1963) famously wrote of the choice to take the less traveled road. The simple yet profound sentiment captures the satisfaction of doing what is right for *you*, rather than simply doing what everyone else does. A common interpretation of these words is that they advocate personal choice—not so much different from the core premise of natural birth!

For all the passionate discussion and even debate about the best way to bring a baby into the world, all sides ultimately want the same outcome: a healthy baby and a healthy mom. It's just that the methods and philosophies to get there can be vastly divergent. Yet they also have interesting intersections, where a choice you make can send you down a path that wasn't quite the one you intended.

Birth Works

Evidence-based data now shows us that women who feel supported and safe during labor and birth have shorter labors, often have more comfortable labors, and have better outcomes than women who are subjected to numerous and endless efforts to micro-manage the birthing process.

> **Oh, Baby!**
>
> Midwife Jenny says: once you pull a laboring woman into the thinking part of her brain, even just by asking her questions and talking to her about what's going on, her hormones change and labor slows. When a woman enters "la-la land," she's in the mammalian part of the brain where the only focus of her being is birthing. She needs to stay there. She's aware of her surroundings; she just can't care about them. All her attention is focused on her body and what it's doing to have the baby. Birthing isn't designed to work well when your brain is going a mile a minute!

No Place Like Home

The less intervention you want, the closer to home you'll want to be. At home, you can direct 100 percent of your effort on your birth without any struggles to reclaim the birthing process. Most natural birth advocates believe home is the most natural place for birth. At a homebirth, there are no bright lights, loud noises, or streams of people rushing in and out. The baby may enter the world into a candlelit room with quiet music playing, or the entire family may be there. The atmosphere is up to you.

Statistics tell us that only a little more than 1 percent of births overall in the United States occur at home. In a few states where legislation and regulation are less restrictive and more supportive of midwifery, the homebirth rate is as high as 5 or 6 percent. Although the percentage is small, the numbers themselves are not. One percent of births means that there are more than 41,000 homebirths in a year. You are not alone if you are considering homebirth!

No Hurry

We sometimes think everything should happen according to some sort of timetable. Many of our daily activities operate this way—work hours, school schedules, and even meal times. We're constantly racing around to get everything done in time. And we carry over the same time-driven logic to pregnancy and birth, from estimating the date of birth to measuring the duration and spacing of contractions. Time becomes the standard by which we determine progress.

Pregnancy and birth don't follow the calendar or the clock. We might think they do, because we use time constructs to measure and discuss pregnancy and birth—nine months (which isn't quite accurate, anyway), six hours, ten centimeters. But pregnancy and birth have their own time frames. The baby initiates labor in its own birth (science tells us the baby sends hormones to the placenta, which in turn sends hormones into the mother's body). We know all kinds of signs that birth is imminent, but we don't really know what determines the start of the birthing process.

We also don't really know how long is too long for the birthing process to take. Within the context of natural birth, birth takes as long as it takes. However, there are clinical data that show an increasing possibility of complications beyond certain time markers. And it is when labor transgresses these boundaries that birth philosophies collide and discussion turns to intervention.

The Intervention Cascade

Birth is an intricate choreography of events that take place in your body, building on one another until the momentum is so in tune and organized that your baby surges into the outside world. One thing leads to six things which in turn lead to dozens of other things—a chain reaction causing a ripple of after-effects. When it comes to birth, there's no such thing as a single intervention. There's no unraveling all that's been done and no going back. With each action, certain events become inevitable; each creates further events that then require more extensive interventions until it's no longer possible for the birth to take any form of a natural path.

Oh, Baby!

In 1965, the first year researchers collected data about the rate of c-sections in the United States, the c-section rate was 4.5 percent. In 2008, the U.S. c-section rate reached 32 percent. And, despite widespread concern and even alarm about the casual use of the surgery, this rate shows no sign of dropping. Even more shocking is that this is not the highest rate in the world. In Brazil's Rio de Janeiro, where surgical birth is the option of choice among women who can afford it, a whopping 89 percent of births are by c-section.

For all procedures, from the seemingly innocuous (such as IVs, hospital gowns, and external fetal monitoring) to the clearly invasive (such as epidural and episiotomy), it's important to weigh the risks and the benefits.

Is C-Section Really an *Option?*

Some doctors consider c-section to be just another option they can offer, pretty much like any other elective surgery. It often comes out sounding something like, "Well, you can tough it out for another who knows how many hours, and we'll just keep a close eye on the baby's heart rate. Maybe things will progress, but maybe you'll need a c-section anyway."

A good number of women accept the offer—they're exhausted, maybe a little scared, and often feeling that it's the best choice. Some women even opt to schedule a surgical birth for whatever reasons are important to them. But a c-section isn't quite the same as a tummy tuck, and a baby's birth really isn't about convenience. Fortunately we're seeing less and less of this in the United States.

Oh, Baby!

Doctors often are more willing to schedule a repeat c-section for a woman who has already had a c-section than to agree to a VBAC (vaginal birth after cesarean section). Yet significant risks come with the c-section package for both mother and baby, which we discuss in Chapter 3.

It's a good idea to have the c-section discussion early on with your practitioner and your partner so there's an understanding in place for the circumstances that may make surgical birth necessary.

Natural Woman

Induced births and repeat c-sections are less likely to take place on weekends than other births, according to data compiled by the U.S. National Center for Health Statistics (NCHS). Nearly three times as many c-sections happen on Tuesday than on Sunday.

What's in a Word?

As you read about natural birth, you may start to think that it's so different that it has its own language. You wouldn't be wrong! Language is very powerful; it's through words that we shape, define, and express our thoughts and emotions.

Think about some of the words you hear when people talk about pregnancy and birth: *delivery*, *labor*, *contractions*, *dilation*, *effacement*, and *childbirth*, to name a few. What images do these words conjure in your mind's eye? Speak these words aloud. How do they sound and feel? Are they maybe a little harsh, sharp, clinical, or even scary?

Now, consider the word "birth." Say it out loud. Feel and hear what a gentle, soft word it is. And what if you say "birthing" instead of "labor"? Sounds a lot nicer, doesn't it? Word associations are potent—capable of activating memories and feelings that in turn initiate hormonal reactions in your body. These reactions either aid or complicate your body's efforts. Wouldn't you rather have surges or waves than contractions? Even now as you're only reading the words, feel the reactions happening within you.

The word "birth" creates a sense of release even as it passes through your lips. It's the tangible as well as spiritual chance to leave behind anything that no longer serves you during this life-altering experience. When you birth your baby, you birth yourself, too—everyone gets a new beginning as you, your partner, and your new baby create, or add to, your family.

The Natural Choice

Imagine what the baby must feel if during labor the mom is screaming and fighting her contractions, afraid of the pain and thinking only about the contractions coming on. We worry a lot about drugs crossing the placenta, but we forget that pretty much *everything* crosses the placenta. Think about the hormones and other chemicals your body releases when you're happy, sad, scared, hungry, calm, or confident. Your baby experiences what you experience.

Your choices shape your baby's first minutes of life outside your body, and these first minutes of life have a good deal to do with how your baby is going to be for the rest of his or her life. Let your baby know, now and every day until your baby's birth, that you're invested in making the birth experience the best it can be.

The Least You Need to Know

- *You* are the person most capable of managing your own birth.

- The first intervention sets in motion a cascade of changes in the birthing process that increasingly limit your ability to influence and shape the birth experience you want to have.

- Knowledge empowers you to make choices and decisions with confidence.

- Although interventions have become so commonplace as to be standard in medical births, there is little evidence to support their routine use.

- The words you choose to talk about pregnancy and birth shape your feelings, expectations, and ultimately your experiences.

Weighing the Risks and Rewards

In This Chapter

♦ The journey of your best birth starts here and now

♦ The path of birth's history

♦ The safety of natural birth today

♦ Trust yourself and your decisions

To hear some people talk, you may think it's less risky to leap from an airplane with a blanket for a parachute than to have a natural birth. Natural birth is not without risks, of course, but neither is medical birth. Very little in life is risk-free. However, you're going to study, take classes, and prepare your body, mind, and spirit—because knowledge and preparation help dissolve the mystery of the unknown.

You're not going to just get up one day, yawn, and scratch your big, beautiful belly and say, "Okay, baby, c'mon out!" You know birth is more—so much more—than this. Being pregnant for the better part of a year gives you time to learn as much as you can about the changes your body's going through and how your baby's growing and developing inside you. Both will culminate in birth before you know it—although right now you may feel like you'll be pregnant forever.

Meanwhile, you have questions. This is good, because the more you know about the process of giving birth, the better prepared you are for you and your baby's birth experience. Whether you have already decided on natural birth or you are still exploring your options, what you learn in this book will help you gain confidence and give you a holistic understanding—a kind of body knowledge—that will center you in labor and guide you as you create a birthing plan.

The Birth You Want

The more you know about the natural birth experience, the more you know about birth. That just makes common sense. You may be coming to this book simply because you are curious but aren't sure whether you have a real desire to have a natural birth. Or maybe there's something more to it than that and your interest is deeper, but you need to know more to make a good decision. Maybe natural birth is appealing because you've "gone organic" in other aspects of your life, and a natural birth seems like a way to validate your trust in Mother Nature. On the flip side, maybe you have enough demands on your time already that you worry whether your lifestyle allows you to commit to the preparation you're pretty sure a natural birth requires.

We understand that choosing natural birth may seem "risky" to you in a lot of senses of that word. Certainly, in our country where most births take place in hospital settings, choosing to have a natural birth (even if it's a natural birth attended by a certified nurse midwife in a hospital birthing center) can seem like you're taking a chance merely by doing something different from what most women are doing. We hope that when you've finished reading this book and are ready to move on to the next book in your stack about pregnancy and birth you will have learned a lot of what you need to know to search your heart and proceed on the course that's right for you.

Naturally, we believe natural birth is a wonderful choice with profound rewards for you and your baby. But we also believe that the birth experience can, and should, *belong* to *you*—and that the more articulately you can express what kind of birth experience you'd like to have and the more willing you are to do the preparation and planning to bring that experience into being, the more likely it is that you'll be ready to own that day you give birth to your baby.

Can You Really Do This?

"Okay, so can I really do this?" This is the biggest question for most women considering a natural birth. And the answer for nearly all women is, yes, *you really can do this*. Your

body and your subconscious mind (the part that functions without your thoughts directing it) know exactly what to do. The exceptions are those women who have medical or other significant factors that bump their pregnancies out of the realm of normal (we talk more about these factors in Chapter 6).

The answer for *you* specifically, however, is perhaps not so straightforward and depends on your beliefs about birth, your faith in the design and function of your body, your partner's support, and your lifestyle. It's important to understand and accept that there are ultimately no wrong answers—whether you choose a natural birth, a medical birth, or a birth experience that's somewhere in between. What matters most is that the choices you make are ones you can commit to and live with.

Pain, fear, and fatigue are the elephants in the room for most women when it comes to considering a natural birth. The biggest question looming in your mind may be, "Will I be strong enough to handle a long, painful labor?" But the real question is, "How will I manage the full range of intense sensations I'll experience while giving birth?" Many people believe a natural, nonmedicated birth is inherently painful. This is not true, and Chapter 4 explains why.

How will *your* natural birth feel? We can't tell you; no one can. Many variables come into play—most significantly, your expectations. What we can tell you is that your body's natural processes are designed to birth your baby, and when allowed to follow those processes, your body releases an astonishing array of chemicals that rival any drug for effectiveness in pain relief, relaxation, and euphoria (yes, euphoria!)—all without harm or side effects for you or your baby.

Oh, Baby!

Studies in recent years suggest a correlation between epidural anesthesia during birthing and the baby having difficulty breastfeeding following birth. Medications that cross the placenta near the time of birth can affect the baby's breastfeeding instinct and sucking patterns, with the baby taking longer to coordinate the necessary movements. Once the baby finally gets started, however, breastfeeding is normal. Epidurals also prolong the second stage of labor so you end up pushing longer.

Can You Make the Commitment?

How long have you been thinking about natural birth? Maybe you and your partner have known since before your pregnancy that you might want to have a natural birth, or maybe you've had a taste of the medical approach to birth and you've decided it doesn't quite fit you. In any case, you've already recognized that you need to educate yourself—and that's the most important step for you to take.

It takes a commitment of time and effort to prepare for *any* birth, natural or medical. Nearly all care providers direct pregnant women to childbirth education classes of some sort because they want you to at least understand the process of birth. Typically, conventional childbirth education classes begin in the second trimester, when your pregnancy is unmistakably real and you're starting to think about things such as diapers, strollers, and taking time off if you're working. You might go to a one-hour class each week for eight weeks, with each class covering a different topic. (Chapter 13 talks about the various kinds of childbirth education.) It may feel a lot like school, and when the classes are over, you may practice your breathing techniques and relaxation methods for a while—but the tendency is to file away the information until the first hint that labor's starting.

Natural Woman

Are you encountering resistance from others to your interest in a natural birth? Sometimes people who are important in your life don't really understand what "natural birth" means, and they don't realize you'll be putting much effort into your preparations. You may consider inviting the person to a class to see what natural birth is really all about.

Preparing for a natural birth takes things to another level. You're not only learning about the processes of birth but also discovering how to work with the flow of those processes to support your body's natural efforts. You have to go beyond the standard "this is the cervix at 10 centimeters" measurement to learn how your body positions influence how quickly and easily your cervix reaches this point of full dilation. When you prepare for a natural birth, you're not only taking classes—you're also taking responsibility for shaping your birthing experience.

You will need to take classes, of course, to learn the methods you can use during labor to keep yourself relaxed and comfortable. These may be entirely new methods for you, such as special breathing techniques (Chapter 13) or hypnosis (Chapter 15). You might turn to familiar practices to use in a specific and focused way during birthing, such as meditation and yoga (as Chapters 10 and 11 discuss). Most importantly, you'll need to practice these methods throughout your pregnancy so when it's time for birthing, they come to you automatically.

Your lifestyle—job, family, and other demands on your time and focus—may or may not support this level of commitment. Does your partner support your interest in a natural birth? This, too, is an important factor when you're looking at making the choice for a natural birth.

What's in It for You?

So you go through all this preparation for a natural birth. What do you get for your time and effort? With a natural birth:

- ◆ You can move around, eat, shower, sit in the birthing tub, and be in any position that makes you comfortable during labor.

- ◆ You can stay naturally hydrated, which is ideal for your body and crucial to optimizing your experience of labor.

- ◆ Your birth unfolds on its own schedule, at its own pace.

- ◆ There are no interruptions or interventions to interfere with your body's normal processes.

- ◆ Your mental focus can stay on your baby and on birthing, without distraction. You can go to that primal place and stay there.

- ◆ You can feel the changes in your body as the time of birth nears so you can push more effectively.

- ◆ Your baby is immediately awake and alert.

- ◆ Your recovery following the birth is likely to be faster and easier.

> **Trusty Midwife Tips**
>
> Once a baby weighs seven pounds, the baby's weight gives better application of the head to the cervix. As well, the baby is stronger and can more easily make the maneuvers, movements, and changes of position needed to make the journey along the birth path. These factors lessen the effort the mother's body must exert to birth the baby.

These are some of the more tangible benefits of a natural birth. For most women, however, one of the greatest rewards of a natural birth is intangible. A natural birth often has that "something extra" that comes from having gone deep within yourself to confront your most primal fears and expectations, and finding that you do indeed have the strength, stamina, and ability to do it.

History's Legacy

If natural birth is so great, then why aren't more women choosing it? It's a complicated question; we need to turn back the pages of history for this answer. But don't worry, there's no test! Of course, women have been giving birth since the beginning of human existence. For the lion's share of this continuum, they have done so without much assistance except from each other. When a woman's "time" drew close, so did the women of her community—her sisters, her women friends, her mother, her grandmother, and often a "wise woman" who knew the secrets of birthing.

This group of women stayed with the laboring woman, helping her to remain comfortable in the familiar surroundings of her own home. One or two may have walked with her while others set up fresh bedding and tidied things a bit. Another may have heated water for a warm bath or made some broth to keep up the birthing woman's strength. The birthing woman was never left alone; someone was always with her for support and encouragement.

The wise woman or another woman in the group served as the midwife to help the baby out and into its mother's waiting arms, to tie off and cut the cord, and to make sure the new mother was clean and warm after the birth. Some of the women then went home—their roles over. Others stayed for a few days after the birth to help with meals and chores, to make sure the baby was nursing, and to take care of the new mom and any other children. This was the way of birth for centuries.

The Invisible Threat of Infection

Until the middle of the twentieth century, a significant risk associated with birth was infection—although no one really understood what this meant. When women became feverish and ill following birth, it seemed an obvious conclusion that somehow the birth was responsible. And so, birth began to acquire a reputation as dangerous.

Doctors became more involved in birthing as an effort to reduce illness. But tragically, doctors were the most common cause of infection with birth. No one yet knew about germs, so there was little hand washing (yuck!). Doctors went from one birth to another, spreading infection from woman to woman. The dreaded illness, from which often there was no recovery, became known as childbed or childbirth fever (*puerperal fever*).

> *Our Baby* **Birthing Book** _____
>
> **Puerperal fever** is a serious bacterial infection that a mother can develop following birth when tissue trauma and cuts provide easy access for bacteria to enter the bloodstream. Puerperal means "around child" and comes from the Latin word *puer*, which means "child."

It eventually became clear that as women increasingly went to doctors, and especially to hospitals, to give birth, more of them became sick—furthering the belief that birth was risky business. Over time, this correlation got turned on its head and the standard became established that pregnancy and birth required medical intervention. The lack of knowledge about infection inseparably fused birth with risk.

Finally, in the 1840s, Hungarian physician Ignaz Semmelweis (1818–1865) made the connection between dirty hands and childbed fever. He noticed that when the doctors in his hospital went from doing autopsies to examining women in labor and delivering babies, their hands were covered in … well, let's just say "debris." So he ordered the students, nurses, and doctors under his jurisdiction to wash their hands in chlorine water. It wasn't so good for the hands, but infection rates plummeted. We now know that routine hand washing has the same effect, so doctors now wash with antibacterial soap instead of chlorine and follow stringent procedures to reduce the risk of infection. And 100 years later, antibiotics came onto the scene. For the most part, the risk of life-threatening infection with birth went away—although the fear associated with birth did not.

Crooked Bodies, Fragmented Design

Rivaling infection as a cause of problems and fear with birthing were bone deformities that made difficult or impossible the baby's passage from the womb. Nutritional deficiencies were the key causes of such deformities, which could twist and contort a woman's skeleton such that she barely had space to accommodate her growing baby or a pelvic opening that would allow the baby to birth. This, of course, meant that sometimes babies got stuck, causing excruciating pain for the woman and often loss of life for the baby (and sometimes for the mother, too).

These kinds of problems, too, became steadfastly bonded with birth—although they really had nothing to do with birth itself. When we look back on this today, it's especially heart-wrenching because we now know how easy it is to prevent the underlying nutritional deficiencies simply through diet. We don't see severe nutritional deficiencies very often in the United States or in other developed countries today because of better nutrition (including fortification of processed grains to ensure adequate vitamin and mineral intake even when your eating habits are less than ideal)—although, as with infection, their legacy lingers.

How Safe, Really, Is Natural Birth Today?

The risks that accompany any kind of birth (except c-sections) are, for most women, so low that they're nearly nonexistent. Most interventions, however, do come with risks ranging from bruising (such as where an IV is placed) to infection. Some of the things that can go wrong, such as the baby attempting to enter the birth path in an awkward position, will happen whether the birth is natural or medical. Other things that can go wrong, such as delays in labor, are often set in motion as a result of intervention rather than from the natural course of birth (the intervention cascade that Chapter 2 discusses).

If a problem arises or something does go wrong during birth, you of course want to have whatever care is necessary and appropriate for the health and well-being of both you and your baby. Your birthing preparation should include specific and detailed discussion with your midwife or doctor so you know what actions your practitioner will take in certain situations. It's important that you trust your practitioner to honor your preferences and desires and also to trust in his or her assessment of a situation so if there truly is a medical emergency, you'll be confident you're receiving the care you need.

Your Health Foundation

There are certain health conditions a woman may have that put her at higher risk for problems during pregnancy as well as birth. Although such health conditions don't necessarily rule out the option of a natural birth, they may influence choices of practitioner and birth location. Health conditions such as uncontrolled diabetes, unresolved high blood pressure (hypertension), kidney disease, and any condition for which you take regular medication may mean you should continue with a doctor's care throughout your pregnancy and for your birth.

Oh, Baby! _____

Having a health condition for which you receive ongoing care and take medications, such as diabetes or high blood pressure, does not necessarily mean a natural birth is out of the question for you. It does mean, however, that you have more questions to ask and that you need to involve the appropriate health-care providers. Make sure all providers who regularly participate in your care know what the others are doing so that everyone is on the same page.

Multiples

Twins are a fairly common variation of normal pregnancy, although in the medical model they bump your pregnancy into the moderate risk category. However, carrying twins does not automatically rule out a natural birth. You'll need to have a practitioner who believes that; the standard approach to multiples is to schedule a c-section. Even if this is a "just-in-case" schedule, it establishes the mind-set for the birth to be surgical. You may need to keep pulling others back toward the birth you envision.

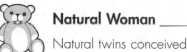

Natural Woman _____

Natural twins conceived without fertility treatments are more common than we think. Three in 100 women conceive twins; the ratio rises with the mother's age to 5 in 100 if she's older than age 35. The chance of having natural higher multiples is much less: 1 in 8,000 for triplets and 1 in 800,000 for quadruplets.

What If You've Previously Had a C-Section?

It has long been the conventional wisdom: once a c-section, always a c-section. However, women and providers alike are challenging this in growing numbers. And for many women whose subsequent pregnancies are normal and healthy, a VBAC (vaginal birth after cesarean) may be much safer than a repeat c-section because of the increased risks associated with surgery. Many women whose pregnancies are otherwise routine and low-risk are able to have a natural birth following a c-section.

Although having had a previous c-section does not in itself rule out a natural birth in a subsequent pregnancy, VBAC remains somewhat controversial. Some providers feel VBAC is appropriate only in a hospital setting, and some oppose it under any circumstances. As with all birthing options, it's important for you to gather full and complete information about your own health situation (including the reason you had a c-section) as well as the risks and benefits of VBAC. Ultimately, each woman's unique circumstances must frame her personal decision.

When Loved Ones Don't Support Your Choices

Sometimes opposition to your plans for a natural birth comes from those you least expect, such as your partner, mom, sister, or best friend since second grade. The more you can learn about pregnancy, birth, and your body, the better equipped you'll be to educate those who don't know how normal birth is.

Some people present more of a challenge. When your husband or partner opposes a natural birth, you might feel frantic or despondent. This is *your* body, and you want to direct the experiences that affect it. But your partner helped create this baby, so how do you now create balance between what each of you wants? Sometimes it's only a matter of uncovering what troubles your partner about natural birth and providing answers that put those concerns to rest.

Maybe your partner or other loved one is afraid that without medical intervention, harm could come to you or the baby, you won't be able to manage the pain or endure the fatigue, or that he or she won't be able to be there for you in the ways that you want.

And the Winner Is ... Your Baby!

Natural birth's rewards for your baby are pretty sweet, too. For starters, your baby enters the world fully awake, alert, and aware. Although those eyes don't see very clearly yet, they do seek you out first. (And isn't it interesting that the baby can see about a foot and half, just about the same distance from your baby at your breast to your face?) After growing, developing, and fine-tuning all those brain synapses in the last weeks of pregnancy, your baby's eager to see who belongs to that voice.

Babies born on their own agendas to secure and confident moms are ready to be in the world. They're relaxed and content, yet alert and aware. The serenity of a natural birth can be disconcerting to those who are used to the usual frenzy of a medical birth, but not to mom and baby, who are both at ease—completely focusing on each other and enjoying this new perspective they now have of each other.

Is it worth all the research and the sifting of information to figure out what you need so you can have your best birth? More and more women (and their partners) are saying, "Yes!"

Feeling Confident About Your Decision

Because you're reading all the information you can find about natural birth and you're talking to women who have had natural births, you're learning that most of what people fear about natural birth is unfounded. Confidence begins to settle within you, and you become assured in your decisions about the kind of birth you want to have.

This confidence goes a long way toward calming other people's fears. Those who object will either realize their concerns are misplaced and they'll come around to support and respect you, or they won't and they'll leave you alone. You can't change what someone else believes. All you can do is stand firm in what *you* believe—and *you* are the one having the baby, after all.

The Least You Need to Know

♦ The more you know about the natural process of birth, the better informed your decisions about *your* birthing experience will be.

♦ Many of the fears and worries we have about natural birth, and birth in general, come from past circumstances that are no longer relevant yet remain woven into the fabric of our beliefs.

♦ Many choices are open to you as you consider the birthing experience you want to have; the more you learn, the better able you are to make informed decisions that you (and others) can trust.

♦ Trust what you learn and what you know.

Part 2

The Truth About Natural Childbirth

For as much as we anticipate with eager joy the arrival of a new baby, there can be a lot of fear and dread surrounding the process of birth itself. How much pain is there, exactly? Is it really possible to experience a natural birth without pain *and* without pain medication? You might be surprised by the real answers! Here's a hint: natural birth is the safest and the most comfortable option for you and your baby when you properly prepare yourself. These five chapters explain why and take an up-close and personal look at birth worries. This material also discusses how to find the right provider to assist with your birth and how to choose the best place for the birth experience you want to have.

Chapter 4

How Much Will It Hurt ... *Really?*

In This Chapter

- Why we believe birth must be painful
- What labor really feels like
- Oxytocin, endorphins, and adrenaline: a powerful hormonal cocktail
- The many ways to stay comfortable during labor and birth
- What you expect is often what you get
- The ecstasy of birth

Birth is likely the most intense experience you'll ever have, but it doesn't have to be the most painful. Pain comes from fear, and fear comes from the unknown. Through your reading and learning, you're going to strip away the unknown. As you find out more, fear will have nowhere to hide and no reason to stick around. Without fear, you can be calm, relaxed, and focused to welcome your baby with joy and love. And here's a little secret we'll let you in on: a natural, nonmedicated birth can be downright orgasmic!

Cultural Origins of Painful Birth

The expectation that birth is not possible without pain is primarily a manifestation of Western culture that's difficult to trace to a clear origin. Once upon a time, normal birth simply happened as part of the birthing woman's daily routine (as it still does in many cultures around the world today). The birthing woman followed her body's guidance for the most comfortable and efficient birthing position and birthed her baby. She then wrapped the baby to keep it warm and dry and carried the baby in a sling as she went about the rest of her day's activities. It was all quite matter-of-fact and, well, routine.

No one really knows what happened to shift expectations so dramatically from a routine to an extraordinary experience. Certainly multiple factors are in play, from the cumulative experience of difficult births to changes in the ways women passed information from one generation to the next as families began to move away from each other.

Even when we look at cultures today where women give birth uneventfully and almost casually, it's not easy to identify tangible reasons for why women's birth experiences are so different. It appears that when the status quo is noninterventionary birth, this becomes the practice as well as the expectation and it greatly shapes the birthing experience for both women and providers. In Holland, for example, more than 80 percent of women birth naturally and without medication or other interventions. Holland also has one of the lowest rates in the world for infant and maternal *morbidity* and *mortality*—the worldwide standard measures of health-care quality and availability.

Birthing Book

Morbidity is the rate of medical conditions that require treatment. **Mortality** is the rate of death.

Cultural and religious beliefs strongly affect our perceptions and expectations surrounding birth. Early belief systems often perceived any form of suffering or pain as evidence of having angered the divine. Surviving the experience indicated that the person somehow managed to achieve appeasement. Even among cultures and religions with disparate views about the relationship between humankind and the divine, similar perceptions developed—many of which persist today. Whether or not you share these beliefs about pain and the divine, they nonetheless pervade Western culture. And from them arises a sense of shame that accompanies natural (and naturally beautiful) functions such as birth (and its conventionally essential predecessor, sex).

Worries and Fears

We all worry. It's part of what makes us human. But for some people, worrying qualifies as a second career. They're always doing it, even when they're doing something else. Mostly, we worry about the unknown and things we can't change. *What if something goes wrong? What if my baby's too big or I'm too small, or my labor fails to progress?*

Well, what if everything goes just like it's supposed to? What if you listen to the messages your body gives you, and all you have to do is go with their flow? What if you feel so great after your baby's birth that you hold her in your arms and dance around the room? Now, these are some of the what-ifs to think about!

It's challenging sometimes to separate the details from the worries. Details are tangible and real, and giving them your attention makes things easier. Worries are intangible and ethereal; like animal shapes in the clouds, they don't really exist except in your imagination. Giving them your attention can make you crazy and perhaps makes those worries more real. Use your mind's eye for a more productive purpose: envision the birth you *want* to have, not the one you fear. A crucial aspect of this is that any kind of worry draws your mind from the positive toward (or outright into) the negative. Deal with real details, yes. But use the awesome power of your mind for positive intent!

So What *Do* You Feel During Labor?

Every person's experience of pain, and every woman's experience of labor, is different. Your experiences can also be very different from one pregnancy to another. "It really didn't hurt!" says Linda about the natural birth of her fourth baby. "It was like bad menstrual cramps or the cramps you get with diarrhea. They call them uterine contractions, but they take over your whole body and they're uncomfortable."

For her natural birth, Linda prepared herself for the birthing experience she wanted to have. She read a lot of books and found a midwife who supported her intentions. "Each time in the hospital, I wasn't going to have drugs—but then I was so uncomfortable I had to have them," Linda says of her first three births. "The labor just went on and on, and I was on my back. With the fourth, I was up on my feet almost all the time or sitting. Then, it was time to give birth. Just a couple pushes and she came out!"

Linda's husband, other kids, and a friend were all at the birth for support and celebration. When she was in labor, Linda ate when and what she wanted and even went with her husband for a walk around a nearby shopping mall when she started feeling bored and restless. After her previous birth experiences, she was amazed how comfortable she felt. "This time there was no episiotomy, everyone was calm, and I was tired but not exhausted. It was entirely different."

Each woman perceives the comforts and discomforts of labor in a unique way. Some women, such as Linda, describe the sensations they feel as being like strong menstrual cramps. Other women describe their experience of labor as waves of pressure or squeezing. Some may use words such as "discomfort" and "uncomfortable"; some women do say labor hurts. The baby's position, the length of labor, the environment, and many other factors influence a woman's ability to relax and work with her body's efforts during birth.

Trusty Midwife Tips

If you feel discomfort or pain during birth, what does your body want to do in response? Not your *brain*, but your body. Does your body want to walk, sway, crouch, or get down on all fours? These are natural reactions to natural messages intended to guide your birthing process. You have to be alert, aware, and unrestricted to engage in them to the fullest.

There is a lot of documentation to support that when a woman prepares well and feels safe, private, unobserved, and unjudged, her experience of discomfort during labor is significantly less. The more you know, the more you can relax and go with the flow of your body's efforts. The more relaxed you stay, the fewer messages of alarm your muscles and tissues send to your brain. When birth is allowed to unfold naturally, in its own time and in a supportive setting, the kind of pain that lives in the common (mis)perception of birth just doesn't exist.

The sensations of birth are unique in that they are productive—they're preparing your body to birth a baby. Part of the issue with pain is our natural tendency to fight it and get away from it or from what's causing it. During labor and birth, these intense sensations send the same kinds of messages—but they're messages intended to guide your body in moving to accommodate the changes that are taking place to let the birth happen. The peak of the contraction lasts only a few seconds; the rest of the time is the build-up to it and the drop from it. Then, there is release and rest until the next one.

Oh, Baby!

Pain medications that bind with opioid receptors in the brain suppress the body's production of natural pain-relieving endorphins.

It's not all about contractions, though. Your body produces an astonishing array of hormones and other biochemicals that change the way your brain interprets messages from nerve receptors. Instead of feeling pain, if you're relaxed and centered in your birthing experience, you feel euphoric. That's not something you'll get from *any* medication.

Your Insensitive Cervix

Your cervix, the muscular gateway between your uterus and the outside world, can't really feel sensation because it has very few sensory nerves (the kinds of nerves that carry messages to your brain). It's not like your fingertips, which have an abundance of sensory nerve receptors. Instead, the cervical nerves are of the kind that tell the cervix what to do—which is basically to contract, expand, or relax—and to pass the same message to the uterus so it can contract or relax, too.

Although your cervix certainly isn't as busy as other muscles (such as, say, your heart), it's not just hanging out in there waiting for your annual pap smear, either. It has things to do. Each month, your cervix expands to allow menstrual flow to leave your body, then contracts and tightens to protect against entry into the uterus.

Your cervix softens, dilates, and moves forward when you ovulate, making it easier to entice sperm to enter. It then moves back toward your sacrum (the fused bones that make up the lowest section of your spine) from the end of your period to when you next ovulate. This is why you might swear your man is suddenly bigger (your cervix is forward and getting banged into during sex), or he got suddenly smaller and you want more of him, deeper (your cervix has moved backward and there is more space). Your cervix also quivers and convulses during orgasm—another effort to draw sperm into your uterus.

Whatever sensations you experience from your cervix's normal activity or from contact, such as during a Pap smear or sex, are indirect. The cervix's movements affect nearby muscles and tissues that do have sensory nerve receptors, and those nerves carry signals to your brain that your brain then interprets as pleasant (orgasm) or not so pleasant (menstrual cramps). How does your brain know which it is? Good question!

To a great extent, it depends on which you believe it is. If you believe you're about to reach orgasm during sex, it's clearly pleasurable. But because we've been told labor hurts—and because the belief that labor hurts is so deeply entrenched in our culture that we take it to be the truth—we expect labor to be painful. So, unless you do something to change that belief within yourself, labor will indeed be painful.

The Myth of the "Pain-Free" Surgical Birth

When your labor is particularly long, the allure of capitulating to a c-section becomes particularly strong. Wouldn't it be great to simply cut to the chase? You wouldn't feel anything more, and then there'd be a baby!

But it's a baby you wouldn't put to your breast for at least several hours, either, and might not even see until then (if you're awake enough yourself). And who knows when you'd be able to raise your baby to your breast by yourself? It may be six weeks at least. That's the typical recovery time during which everything, from peeing to picking up your baby, hurts (and heaven help you if you sneeze or cough).

A c-section, when it's truly necessary for your baby's or your own health and well-being, is a great and wonderful thing. But it's not the ticket to a pain-free birth. Its trade-off value diminishes when the circumstances are more about convenience. Being tired is not a health risk! A natural labor and birth are far less painful, in the end, than a c-section—not to mention better overall for both you and your baby.

Those Wonderful Birth Hormones

Hormones are the centerpiece of fertility. They regulate sex, ovulation, conception, pregnancy, birth, and lactation—and, as most women know, the desperate need for chocolate! As your body's chemical messengers, your hormones direct just about every other function of your body, too, although we'll focus only on the hormones of birth here.

There are four major players: oxytocin, endorphins, adrenaline, and prolactin. We'll talk about the first three in this chapter, and we'll get to prolactin in Chapter 21 (it takes center stage with breastfeeding).

Oxytocin: Can You Feel the Love?

Oxytocin is where it all starts. Two glands buried in the center of your brain produce and store oxytocin: the hypothalamus makes it, and the pituitary gland holds it. Oxytocin is often called the hormone of love; it makes us feel all warm and fuzzy, setting the stage for sex.

We might also call it the surging hormone: the pituitary gland sends oxytocin into the bloodstream in surges to participate in ejaculation in men, orgasm in both men and women, and, of course, labor and birthing. In birthing, the pituitary releases increasingly larger and more frequent surges of oxytocin. The oxytocin acts on special cells in the wall of the uterus, called oxytocin receptors, to progressively intensify the uterus's rhythmic contractions.

Synthetic oxytocin (the drug Pitocin) is designed to act on the same receptors in the body as its natural counterpart; doctors may use it to induce or stimulate uterine contractions during labor. Although Pitocin causes many of the same actions as natural oxytocin, it doesn't have the same overall effects. Pitocin overrides the body's natural oxytocin and does not trigger the release of endorphins. So endorphin and oxytocin production drops way off.

With endorphins, the body's natural pain relievers, knocked out of the picture, more intense pain is just waiting to take over—so pain medications are nearly always necessary. It becomes a downward spiral, and eventually the body's own hormones become so suppressed that they're ineffective. When this happens, the intervention cascade is underway and it's very difficult to recover the natural process.

> **Trusty Midwife Tips**
>
> Your baby produces oxytocin during birth, too. Scientists believe it's the baby's oxytocin output that initiates labor. Oxytocin also aids mother-baby bonding at birth and encourages breastfeeding.

Endorphins: What a Rush!

Endorphins (which are natural opiates, as in opium) are the feel-good chemicals your body releases in response to certain kinds of physical stress. Think "runner's rush" and you have the right idea—that flood of "I can do anything" that surges through you just when you hit the point where you think you can't run any faster, farther, or longer.

Endorphins are often called nature's pain relievers. They bind with opioid receptors in your brain—the same specialized nerve endings that pain-relieving medications such as meperidine (Demerol) and morphine attach to. This binding produces a great "ahh" response in your brain, shutting off pain messages that the nerves are channeling to your brain. At the same time, endorphins also help you feel alert and acutely attuned with all that's happening in your birth process.

During birth, your body begins producing endorphins in response to the high levels of oxytocin circulating through your system. It's like a loop: the oxytocin triggers the endorphins, and then the pituitary gland releases more oxytocin. This lovely cycle, which gains momentum through the second stage of birthing (which culminates in your baby's birth), is what we might call the "birthing high."

When those endorphins release and start coursing through your system, your baby feels them, too. Your baby knows it's time to be born, and it's a welcome, anticipated event. Along with being exhilarating, endorphins are also relaxing—which allows the baby to come down the birth path quicker and in a better position.

Adrenaline: Hey, Baby ... Let's Go!

Adrenaline (also called epinephrine) is your body's "let's go!" hormone. It's the cornerstone of the fight-or-flight response. Anxiety makes your body ready to fight or flee. Your body pours on the adrenaline, pumping up your heart rate and blood pressure and sending more blood to the muscles that move you. Adrenaline wants you to get outta there, right now!

Now, adrenaline has great purpose when you do need to get out of harm's way—and also when you're ready to push out your baby. In birthing's second stage, after your cervix has thinned and opened (effaced and dilated, to be technical), your adrenaline surges. This is the signal for your body to move. The urge to get up is intense. You may want to pace, twist, bend, squat—anything to get moving. This is your body's way of getting gravity involved in the process. That boost of adrenaline is the hallmark of *transition*, the point at which the efforts of labor shift from opening and thinning your cervix to pushing the baby out.

> **Birthing Book**
>
> **Transition** is the phase of labor at which effort switches from preparing your body for birthing to the process of moving the baby along the birth path.

In the ideal natural birth, the birth itself is almost anticlimactic. You're calm, low-key, and maybe even asleep. You're not at all distressed about pain or anything else. Someone looking in on the scene might perceive that there's nothing at all going on—certainly not a birth. When your body's ready, the adrenaline surge gets you a little agitated—you walk around for a bit, then there are a few strong surges, and the baby comes out.

As soon as you're not calm, however, things hurt. When your anxiety builds, your body cranks up the adrenaline. And when your body is pouring out the adrenaline, it can't generate oxytocin. So as the adrenaline goes up, the oxytocin and endorphins go down. The birthing process slows and may even stop. The baby feels the adrenaline, too, and also becomes agitated. Adrenaline increases both your and your baby's heart rate. If you're in a hospital or birthing center with fetal monitoring, it's easy for staff to determine at this point that the baby is in stress (it is, in the short term) and that you need intervention (you probably don't, yet).

You can reclaim the natural actions of your body's birthing hormones by calming yourself and focusing your thoughts to be positive and supportive for your birthing. When you feel agitated, get up and walk. This is what your body wants you to do, and it will help restore the birthing hormones. Remind yourself that you can do it! Once your confidence returns, so does your sense of comfort and purpose.

The Power of Expectation

Your brain perceives sensory input—messages that sensory nerves carry from all parts of your body—as pleasure or pain according to a framework of stored interpretations. We're pre-programmed with some of these interpretations from a survival basis. Events such as grabbing a hot pan from the oven without a mitt or slicing a finger instead of a tomato generate the "can't-get-away-fast-enough" response. Most everything else we learn, either through our own experiences or through the stories and warnings we hear from other people.

Think Positively—It's No Cliché

All too often we focus on what we *don't* want rather than on what we *do* want. When you're thinking about your birth experience, you may say that you don't want an epidural, you don't want pain medication, and/or you don't want a c-section. While this may all be true, consider the shift in your thought processes and how you feel about the birth when you say instead:

- ◆ "I know my body is fully capable of stretching and relaxing to allow gentle passage for my baby, and I trust in my body's ability to give birth."

- ◆ "I have many methods available to me to remain calm and comfortable during labor and birth, and I trust in my ability to use them."

- ◆ "I embrace the birthing process and the power I have within myself, as a woman, to birth my baby with focus, intent, and joy."

Also, stay in the company of like minds! Avoid TV shows and movies that present birth as hard and painful. Don't listen to the stories of women who want to tell you how awful their birth experiences were. You don't need that. Instead, seek women who have had natural birth, especially homebirth, and encourage them to talk about water birth, hypnosis, breathing, and other methods for improving comfort during labor and birth. Theirs are the stories you want to know!

This, Too, Shall Pass

Labor is not like stubbing your toe or twisting your ankle. There's no sudden, unrelenting pain. Contractions build, peak, and then release. The most intense part of a contraction lasts five or six seconds, then you may have up to five or six minutes of down time to relax until near the end of your labor, when your down time might only be a minute or two. But when you reach that point, you know you're almost finished and your focus shifts. If you're tense and scared, though, you won't be able to let yourself settle into the calm between the peaks—and before long your labor will feel relentless.

> **Birthing Book**
>
> **Dilation** refers to the size of the cervical opening. **Effacement** is the thinning and stretching of the cervix. Dilation and effacement are the key medical measures of labor's progression and must occur for vaginal birth to take place.

Many times, the outward focus on birth tends to be rather narrow and organ-specific. "What's the cervix doing … do we have *dilation* and *effacement*? How long and far apart are contractions?" When your uterus takes over in labor, every structure in your body knows it. Many of those structures have their own roles to play, so they're busy with that. Others don't have anything to do but get excited because they're right there, so they tense, too. Then, you get tense all over because your muscles are tight—and tight muscles hurt. It becomes a nonproductive cycle.

Grantly Dick-Read, the British obstetrician known today as the father of childbirth education, picked up on the correlations among these factors—fear, tension, and pain—and recognized that preventing, or at the very least interrupting, the cycle was crucial to a woman's comfort during birth. From his observations arose the first structured approach to educating women about breathing, relaxation techniques, and birth. Others followed with variations on the concept, all with the same goal of maintaining calm, control, and confidence. Chapter 13 details the most common of these techniques.

Methods to Maintain Your Comfort

There are so many ways you can help yourself stay comfortable during birthing. The only limit is your imagination. This is a great time to be thinking outside the box—to go beyond convention. Listen to your body. What do you feel like doing? Most of the time, that's the best thing for you to do.

Water, walking, dancing, and singing all relax both body and mind, letting the birth hormones prepare you for birthing. Feel like making love? Go for it! (As long as your membranes are intact.) It's nature's best way to relax and get even more of those hormones flowing. Have your partner massage tight muscles, dance with you, and support you so you can get in the positions that are most comfortable.

Gravity is your best friend during labor. It pulls the baby onto the cervix, which further stimulates the release of oxytocin, which opens and thins the cervix. Your entire pelvic structure is working to realign itself for this grand event—your hips are widening from side to side, and your pubic bone is shifting forward. Your sacrum (tailbone) moves farther back. It's a lot harder for all this to happen when you're lying flat on your back.

Oh, Baby!

> The typical reason for women to be on their backs during birth is that it makes it easier for the doctor to see what's happening. This isn't an approach that makes birthing easier for the woman, however. A recent study showed that women who birth in an upright position have less pain and shortened labor, although they do experience slightly more tissue trauma and blood loss.

Water is especially soothing and calming during labor. When you can submerge most of your body in water, the water removes 75 percent of the feeling of gravity. All the effects of labor still happen, but they just don't hurt. Water helps you relax, which opens your chest so you can breathe deeply and get more oxygen to you and to your baby. And what's not to enjoy about floating in warm water? It's very primal itself, connecting you with your baby who's floating inside you.

Hypnosis is another highly effective method you can use to get beyond your fears to focus on the birthing experience you want. There's a common belief that birth by hypnosis means loss of conscious awareness of what's happening with your birthing, but this is—like so many common beliefs about birth—simply not true. Hypnosis is all about focusing on what you *do* want rather than what you *don't* want. We just want to introduce these methods here; the chapters in Part 4 talk about the methods in greater detail.

Here are some of the many ways you can improve your comfort during labor and birthing. Some are things to lay a good foundation, and others are methods to use as you need them.

- Knowledge about what's happening
- Good nutrition throughout your pregnancy
- Being in water: bathtub, shower, birth tub
- Movement: changing positions, walking, squatting
- Listening to your intuition
- Acupressure
- Craniosacral massage
- Support and encouragement from your partner
- Massage
- Hypnosis
- Homeopathy
- Essential oils
- Herbs and herbal teas
- Singing and vocalization
- Cuddling and smooching (Ina May Gaskin's favorite—and usually the dad's, too!)
- Visualization
- Birth ball
- Loving touch
- Eating and drinking to stay nourished and hydrated
- Anything you can imagine to help you feel better

Orgasmic Birth

If you thought birth was like orgasm, wouldn't you rush to sign up? But no one ever says in a childbirth education class, "Hey, folks, listen up: orgasm and birthing are basically the same process." And no one ever says, "Whoa, that orgasm was the most painful experience of my life." Culturally, we've separated birth from its sexual beginnings. We want birth to be about cute little bundles of joy, not about the passionate union of the bodies and souls that created a new life.

Yet it happens, more often than you hear about, that these two experiences intersect and a woman has an orgasm during birthing. Birth, like sex, is intimate, intense, ecstatic, and powerful. When your partner, your baby's father, shares the experience of birth with you in the same passion he shared during the love making, what could be more beautiful? Now there's a revolutionary concept: expect birth to be as ecstatic and joyful as sex!

What Does Birth Feel Like to Your Baby?

If the experience of birth is so intense for you, how does it feel to your baby? Observations of the baby's activities during birth tell us that the baby is not just along for the ride. In a natural, nonmedicated birth the baby is alert and aware—an active participant in birthing who turns and twists, flexes and tucks, and maneuvers around to get into position for his or her easiest movement through the birth path. (Conversely, in a medicated birth the baby, like the mother, is groggy, disoriented, and passive.)

As a fully sentient being, your baby feels the pressure of your body's effort. Because he or she is naturally relaxed and supple, your baby has no reason to interpret these sensations as pain. Your baby hears the sounds of your body—your heartbeat, the activities of digestion, the air entering and leaving your lungs, and your voice. He or she also hears sounds beyond your body, such as conversation and music. Your baby will be listening for your voice when he emerges—after all, he's been hearing it for quite some time and knows it well. For your baby, a natural, relaxed, nonmedicated birth is a welcome and pleasant event. Your baby is eager to meet you!

The Least You Need to Know

- A natural, nonmedicated birth does not have to hurt.
- Your body produces powerful hormones during birthing that, when you're relaxed and calm, can not only relieve discomfort but actually give you a feeling of euphoria.
- Moving around and staying upright during your labor allows gravity to help your baby maneuver into position and helps your body prepare itself for birth.
- Your expectations are the strongest influence that shapes your birthing experience.
- Orgasmic birth is not only possible but much more common than you realize.
- Your baby fully participates in a natural, nonmedicated birth and arrives in the world alert and aware.

Chapter 5

Is Your Body in Shape for a Natural Birth?

In This Chapter

- ◆ Your body already has the perfect design for a natural birth
- ◆ Swim (or just float around in the water)
- ◆ Walk and talk with your partner while you're still two
- ◆ Meeting your baby's and your own needs; it's about nutrition, not weight

You want the best for your baby and yourself, naturally, during your pregnancy and birth. Is your body ready for this grand adventure? To prepare for a natural birth, you may need to make some changes in your lifestyle to support a healthy pregnancy (and you're probably already doing that).

As with any significant physical undertaking, you want to be as strong and healthy as possible for a natural birth. You'll want to improve your flexibility, if you can, and learn breathing techniques that help you focus and relax as well as get more oxygen into your bloodstream during birthing.

Your Natural Body Is in Perfect Shape!

Your body is in great shape for a natural birth because you're a woman, and this is what your body's designed to do. A natural birth happens between your ears as much as anything. It's more about your mindset and what you believe, not how many sit-ups you can do or how often you go to the gym. That's why we encourage you to learn as much as you can about pregnancy and birth. If you feel like you have to "get fit" to birth a baby, it implies your body's not ready and that's not true.

What *can* make you out of shape for a natural birth, however, are other factors that we don't usually associate with fitness: inadequate nutrition, dehydration, and feeling fear, guilt, and doubt. Unfortunately, these factors often arise from efforts to get fit for birth … when you start to say to yourself, "I'm pregnant now, and I should be in better shape." So we say to you, "Enough with the judgment already!"

Your Body Knows What Shape to Be In

Your body begins to get in shape for birthing from the moment of conception. Even before you know you're pregnant, your body's already changing. Hormones begin surging through your body, busily directing the re-sculpting that will take place over the 40 weeks or so that your baby will live and grow within you. Ligaments and muscles soften so they can stretch to accommodate your expanding belly. Blood volume increases. Your breasts enlarge.

> **Natural Woman** _____
>
> "But these aren't big enough to feed a baby!" Women often bemoan small breasts as inadequate for their intended purpose. But what you see is not necessarily what you get. Large breasts do not automatically produce more milk, overall, than small breasts. Your breasts will make exactly the right amount of milk to nourish and satisfy your baby.

Every part of your body changes in some way to participate in this joyous event— all without any conscious effort or even thought on your part. You may feel like you should have greater control over the changes that are taking place, but nature has you covered on this one.

Stay Active!

There are things you can do to improve your body's capabilities without stressing out or feeling like you just want to trade in your current body for a new model.

Life doesn't work that way; you have to make the best of what you have. And you have more going for you than you realize; it's always easier, for some reason, to focus on what we want to change rather than what we have going for us—and that others might even envy. Now, that's a different way to look at things, isn't it? But it's true. We're all too quick to let our perceived shortcomings stop us before we even try, although we seldom see our own strengths and assets for the capabilities they give us.

You don't need to join a gym or take up step aerobics (although if you already have an exercise routine, great!), but do stay active. For most women, whatever you do routinely is usually fine. Just listen to your body. Your loosening and relaxing ligaments and joints may create some challenges, especially later in your pregnancy. You may need to walk instead of run or swim instead of go to your aerobic dance class. Do you warm up before and warm down after an activity session (even walking)? Warming up before activity sends the message to your muscles and joints that it's time to pay attention—which they're eager to do. And warming down after activity is a way to let your body ease gently back to its normal state—and to thank those muscles and joints for giving you such a satisfying and productive workout.

Generally, if you feel better after the activity, you're doing fine. But if you find yourself feeling tired or even dreading it, cut back or take a break. Talk to your midwife or doctor if you feel that exercise you'd normally do as a matter of course is proving difficult or painful. And make sure you replenish your calories—especially protein—and fluids. (Chapter 9 gets into the details of nutrition and hydration.) The baby takes what it needs off the top, so you end up on the short end if you cheat yourself on food, water, or sleep. Sometimes you may feel fine right after exercising but have trouble sleeping or find yourself dragging the next day. These are signs that you're doing too much or not getting enough calories and fluids.

> **Oh, Baby!**
>
> Dehydration is the enemy of natural birth. Your tissues cannot stretch as they're capable of doing, and as they need to, without adequate fluid. So drink lots of water—not soda, tea, coffee, or even juice—but good, old-fashioned water. This is important throughout your pregnancy, and it prevents swelling, too!

If your lifestyle is already active, stay with it as long as it makes you feel better—not worse. You may need to sideline some activities as your pregnancy advances: bicycling, horseback riding, skating, skiing, snowboarding, intense running, racquet sports, and team sports where contact is likely (such as soccer, basketball, and volleyball). Your balance, coordination, and agility naturally shift as your belly expands.

Whatever you do that gets you moving is good for you and for your baby. Maybe you walk three miles every day at lunch, or simply walk from your car to your front door. The more the better, of course (within reason). Just stick with it. Getting outdoors in the fresh air is good for you, and walking is one of the most efficient and effective activities for overall good health. Each cell in your body appreciates every step you take.

Low-Stress Ways to Stay Fit for Birthing

Activity	Benefit
Walking	Improves aerobics; strengthens leg and core abdominal muscles; provides a break from your regular activities; helps maintain healthy weight; easy and free to do; can do it anywhere; great opportunity to spend quality time with your partner
Swimming	Strengthens and tones all muscle groups; great aerobic workout; improves breath control and rhythm; eliminates effects of gravity; no worries about balance; soothing and relaxing to be in the water
Dancing	Improves flexibility; helps you "tune in" to your body; can do it by yourself or with your partner; music can be calming; rhythmic movements are soothing to your baby
Low-impact aerobics	Great workout for your heart and lungs; strengthens and tones all muscles in your body; encourages new bone growth; improves balance and coordination; provides social interaction if done in a class setting
Yoga	Improves flexibility, balance, and breath control; meditative aspect is relaxing and stress-reducing; encourages connection between body, mind, and spirit; can do alone or with a group
Tai Chi	Improves flexibility, balance, and breath control; can provide a social experience if done with a group; helps you learn to work with your body's energy as well as physical abilities; can have a meditative aspect

Water Workout

Swimming and water aerobics are great activities during pregnancy. In the water, you can feel nearly weightless, which takes the pressure off your joints and muscles. There are no awkward balance issues when you're in the water, either. You can move and feel like you're not even pregnant. Swimming also builds your aerobic capacity, putting more oxygen into your blood with every breath. You'll appreciate this now, as your stamina increases with regular aerobic exercise, and later during the birth process when your body's demand for oxygen intensifies.

Trusty Midwife Tips

Another advantage to enjoying activities in the water, such as swimming and water aerobics, is that it lets you experience how the water might affect your body should you be interested in using a birthing tub during labor. (Chapter 14 discusses water birth.) You can feel how water relieves the pressure of gravity, especially later in your pregnancy.

It's All in the Way You Carry Yourself

The best class you can take when you're pregnant is yoga. Yoga strengthens and tones your muscles, extends your flexibility, calms your mind, and teaches you to focus on your breath. It also teaches you how to be still and to be relaxed in your body, which are invaluable skills during birth. Yoga is also something you can do by yourself throughout your pregnancy.

If you take a yoga class, try to find a teacher who has experience working with pregnant women and who knows how to modify the poses to accommodate your shifting center of gravity. Chapter 10 discusses yoga in detail.

Trusty Midwife Tips

Midwife Jenny encourages women to hold hands as you walk with your partner, especially if this is your first baby—because this is the last time you'll be a couple (baby makes three!). It also gives the two of you a chance to talk. Some people are more likely to open up when they're doing something else such as walking, and feel more free to open up about their worries and fears when they can approach them somewhat sideways and in a nonthreatening setting.

The Matter of Weight

You're going to gain weight with this baby, and that's a very good thing. Some of the added weight is yours, reflecting the changes in your body to accommodate this life growing within it. For example, your blood volume increases by half—talk about water weight! Your uterus is growing, too. Your body also wants to increase its fat stores because it's stockpiling energy just in case you need it. You have to go with the flow of that one; it's part of the grand design that makes your body so perfect for bringing forth new life. And remember that some of the added weight comes from your baby and placenta.

But how much weight *should* you gain? Every woman considers this, and many women anguish over it. Are you gaining enough? Are you gaining too much? How do you know, and how do you maintain the right balance? Weight is a touchy subject in pregnancy and gets a lot of attention from a medical perspective, with concerns about the potential of increased risk for complications such as preeclampsia and *gestational diabetes*.

Birthing Book _____

Gestational diabetes is the development of insulin resistance (an inefficiency in the way the body handles insulin) or diabetes during pregnancy. Gestational diabetes may require insulin or oral medication, although the body usually corrects itself after birthing.

Healthy eating, with an emphasis on increasing the amounts of protein and reducing the amounts of sugar you eat, is a good strategy no matter your weight. There's some evidence that keeping your body in the proper nutritional balance reduces your risk for preeclampsia and gestational diabetes.

Overweight women have babies all the time, though, just like everybody else. Women of all shapes and sizes have been birthing successfully since the beginning of human existence. It's important to keep coming back to this fact as your touchstone when self-doubt and fear overcome you. Pregnancy is not the time to worry about, or try to address, weight concerns if they exist for you! Your mission—your *only* mission—is to provide as healthy and safe an environment as possible for your growing baby and for yourself.

You do the best for both of you when you set aside any and all concerns about weight and instead turn your attention toward eating nutritiously, drinking plenty of water, and getting some daily activity. If you eat healthful food, you will gain exactly what you need to gain to make a healthy baby. The weight gain charts have no idea what *you* need. Focusing solely on weight can raise doubt about your ability to have the birth you desire. Instead of getting caught up in perceptions about what you can't do and what might go wrong, put your attention on the many things you can do and that will go right in your birthing experience.

Eat Well, Eat Often

You have to eat when you're pregnant. You're supplying the nutrition for the baby growing within you. Whatever your diet doesn't provide, the baby will take from your own nutrient stores. If you're not replenishing these stockpiles, however, before long you're going to feel the drain.

Don't be thinking, "I'll be tight with calories until my eighth month so I don't gain too much weight." By the eighth month, your baby's nearly done! The early weeks, when your baby's basic body systems (including her brain) are first developing, are especially crucial when it comes to nutrition. Fitness is about nutrition, too. Your weight gain during pregnancy is not about getting fat; you're making an entirely new human being from scratch.

Oh, Baby! _____

You can toss that gold standard for assessing health and weight—body mass index (BMI)—right out the window when you're pregnant. And you really don't want to be looking at your weight as something that's on a chart. If you want to look at a chart, cruise through the food pyramid. This can help you choose new and nutritious foods to meet the needs of your body and your baby, and to maintain a healthy nutritional balance.

So eat often during the day—small amounts, not bigger platefuls—and eat well. Graze. Eat when you're hungry, and eat what appeals to you. If ice cream and chocolate become your main food groups, though, you'll have to force yourself to branch out. Have a steak, beef, or salmon; your baby needs the protein. Your protein requirement increases by a third during pregnancy. Do you eat a vegetarian diet? Eat about a third more of your usual proteins—healthful choices include legumes, whole grains and whole grain products, seeds, and nuts (though beware the oil and salt with these). Hummus, too, is a nutritious and tasty treat. And you certainly don't have to eat vegetarian to enjoy plant-based proteins!

> **Trusty Midwife Tips** _____
>
> A good prenatal vitamin is something you should take during your pregnancy, especially for the calcium, magnesium, and vitamin D—the building blocks of healthy bones. This is important because your baby is drawing from your calcium stores (your bones), and many women tend to have marginal calcium levels themselves as milk has fallen by the wayside in the modern daily diet. Folic acid (also called folate), which all prenatal vitamins include, is crucial to support your baby's developing brain and nervous system, and specifically to prevent neural tube defects. Ideally, you should begin taking a prenatal vitamin before you get pregnant, and certainly just as soon as you discover that you are pregnant.

How's Your Health?

Sometimes there are health concerns that affect your desire for a natural birth. Most of the time, you can work with your health issues as long as you have a fully supportive care provider and fully understand how your particular health situation affects your pregnancy and birthing. Once again, remember that your body was designed to carry and birth a baby. There are many, many variations on that design, and more than 90 percent of those designs work just fine to give birth without any outside meddling.

Health Conditions

Some underlying health conditions may affect the course of your pregnancy and birthing—notably, hypertension and diabetes for which you regularly take medications. Such conditions do not inherently preclude natural birth, however. Generally, if your health permits you to become pregnant, it also will support a natural birth. You just sometimes have to search a little harder to find a care provider who supports your desire for a natural birth.

If you have a health condition that's under control with medication, you'll want to work with your care provider to make any necessary dosage or other adjustments as your pregnancy advances so your condition remains stable. Your provider may want to see you more frequently to keep tabs on your condition. If you're seeing one provider for your regular health care and a different provider for care during pregnancy and birth (which many women do), you'll want to make sure each knows what the other is doing to help keep you healthy and strong.

Trusty Midwife Tips

Not so long ago, lifestyle itself was a key danger in pregnancy and birthing. Women lacked vital nutrition, leading to diseases such as rickets that caused deformities of the bones (including the pelvis). Babies did get stuck during birth because their mothers' bodies were structurally unable to allow their passage. Today, we don't see these diseases and their problems in developed countries, although they remain a concern in some parts of the world.

Health Risks

Remember that what goes into your body goes into your baby's body, too. Don't let this make you crazy, but do think about it. Smoking, drinking, and drugs are of course all usual suspects headlining the list when it comes to things you really should avoid. With cigarette smoking, this includes exposure that comes from being around people who smoke.

Products you may ordinarily take without a second thought could have important and sometimes less-than-pleasant side effects in pregnancy. Talk with your care provider if you have any concerns about products—such as herbs and botanicals or over-the-counter medications—you've been taking or want to take.

However, be aware that the more medically oriented your care provider is, the less likely he or she has a lot of knowledge about herbals; that's just not much a part of conventional medicine. You can call or visit (to consult) a local midwife who uses herbs, and there are lots of good midwifery resources online.

No matter your shape or size, when you look in the mirror, what you see is the miracle of creation. Another life is preparing to enter the world, and your body is the vessel that contains, loves, and nourishes it. What could be more beautiful?

Natural Woman

"When you've had children, your body changes; there's history to it. I like the evolution of that history; I'm fortunate to be with somebody who likes the evolution of that history. I think it's important to not eradicate it. I look at someone's face and I see the work before I see the person. I personally don't think people look better when they [have cosmetic procedures]; they just look different. You're certainly not staving off the inevitable. And if you're doing it out of fear, that fear's still going to be seen through your eyes. The windows to your soul, they say."

—Cate Blanchett, Australian actress and mother of three, in *Vanity Fair*

The Least You Need to Know

◆ Daily physical activity helps your body stay strong, flexible, and capable for a natural birth.

◆ If you're already a gym rat, it's okay to keep at it as long as you feel better, not worse, with your level of activity.

◆ It's important to replenish the calories and fluids you use during exercise with nutritious foods and plenty of water.

◆ What's more important than how much weight you gain during your pregnancy is that what you eat provides good nutrition for you and for your growing baby.

Is a Natural Birth Dangerous?

In This Chapter

- How we came to perceive birth as dangerous
- The urge to want to "fix" everything, even when things are going just fine
- The not-so-hidden agenda that can drive intervention
- Situations that do warrant concern

By the time your belly expands enough for other people to exclaim, "Oh! You're pregnant!" instead of waiting for you to bring it up, you have quite a relationship going with your baby. You probably talk and maybe sing or read to your baby already. You know whether your baby's a night owl or an early bird, a swimmer or a floater, bobbing into your diaphragm or bouncing on your bladder.

And you probably have just a little (or maybe more than a little) anxiety dancing around in your thoughts. Are you doing all you can to have a wonderful birthing experience? Is it going to hurt your baby—or you—to let the birth unfold at its own pace, if that pace differs from what convention holds to be "normal"? How will you know that everything's really okay?

You want to fully experience a joyous birth without outside interference or constraints. So let's take a look at the worries and fears and separate them from the reality of the natural birth experience you can—and are entitled to—have.

Everybody Worries

You're making a lot of decisions with intent rather than by default when you're planning a natural birth, which is empowering—although it can also be a little scary. When you do things the way "everybody" does them, it's easy to have confidence in your decisions because they're not really your decisions—you're only following "everybody" else.

Well, sometimes everybody is wrong. Look how long everybody believed Earth was flat before anyone actually checked it out! We draw conclusions from what we know, which is sometimes limited. When we learn more, often the original conclusions change. Once the facts are out in the open for everybody to see, the tide of opinion begins to change. Admittedly, that tide can move at a snail's pace, and some people hold on to old ideas and beliefs despite evidence that disproves them.

So it is with natural birth (and especially natural birth at home). The numbers say it all: natural birth and homebirth are just as safe as hospital birth. But because most women give birth in hospitals with medical interventions to "help" things along, the belief remains entrenched that birthing in any other way is inherently unsafe. Like Earth being flat, this is simply not true.

Birth's Mythology of Danger

If birth is such a beautiful and natural process, why does the perception of it as dangerous so fully shroud it such that we've come to dread the process? We're willing to go *through* it for its outcome—a baby—but only because there's no other way (the speculation of science fiction aside). Within the psychology of it, this duality is like the exaggerated fear of being in an airplane crash. Millions of people fly safely every day, yet even the most experienced flier feels that twinge of uncertainty when the plane hits takeoff speed at the end of the runway. As with air flight, the facts of birth don't support the reality. Millions of babies are born each year, safe and healthy.

All the fretting and worrying about the danger of birth comes from long-past history (as Chapter 1 discusses), not modern reality. But that danger has become part of the mythology surrounding birth—now so deeply imbued in our perceptions that it has created its own false reality—that it has spawned an entire metaphorical literary tradition in which the creative power of pushing new life into the world comes at great peril to the woman who bears it. From fairy tales and myths to Frederic's beloved Catherine in Ernest Hemmingway's *A Farewell to Arms* to Gertie in the J-Lo and Ben Affleck chick-flick *Jersey Girl*, crisis and even death while giving birth are good drama.

> **Natural Woman**
>
> A girl born in 1800 had a life expectancy of 40 years; a boy, 35 years. Even with the "dangers" of birth, women lived longer than men! Life itself, not birthing, was dangerous. And it's in living where we've made the great advances that set the stage for all else: a girl born in 2008 can expect to live to eventually confront 80 candles on her birthday cake (a boy, 78).

When the Numbers Do the Talking

Thanks to much-improved practices and knowledge, along with antibiotics and technology, the birth experience has become very safe for both mothers and babies—especially birth in a hospital, which remains the location where most births occur. Fewer than 1 in 11,000 women in the United States die while giving birth today, and most of these deaths are from complications resulting from interventions such as c-section or occur in high-risk pregnancies.

Now that there are enough women opting for natural birth at home to attract the attention of statisticians, reports are starting to come out that demonstrate the safety of planned natural birth at home with the assistance of a licensed, certified, or nurse midwife. Deaths (mother or baby) are no more common than with births taking place in a hospital. Complications, however, are significantly fewer in homebirths because interventions are significantly fewer.

The numbers that continue to rise, alarmingly, are of complications related to hospital birth interventions—so much so that lowering them is a main objective of *Healthy People 2010*, the U.S. initiative to improve the overall health of the American population. Nearly one third of women who birth in the hospital experience complications requiring treatment of some kind (such as infection and adverse drug reactions); *Healthy People 2010* aims to reduce this rate by one third by the year 2010.

Birth Is Safe ... It's Intervention That's the Danger

Today, birth is the leading reason why women of childbearing age are admitted to the hospital—and more than three million of them are admitted each year in the United States. That's not such a big deal. The hospital can be a fine place for birthing your baby (as long as you have compassionate doctors, good nurses, skilled midwives, and strong advocates to look out for your desires and best interests). Many hospitals have gone to great lengths to establish birthing units that are less institutional. But a hospital is a hospital; its mission is to care for those who are ill.

Natural Woman

In the early 1900s, about 1 in 1,400 births in the United States resulted in the death of the mother. By then, anesthesia had become the siren song of the medical model for birth, but sterile technique was still rather crude and antibiotics were newly discovered. Infection and hemorrhage resulting from misguided medical meddling were common life-threatening dangers confronting every woman who opted for a hospital birth. Today, a century later, about 1 in 11,000 births results in the mother's death—a vast improvement.

The birthing unit is the only location in a hospital where those admitted are well and healthy. The cheerily decorated doors are no barrier to germs, though. Those germs—many of which do not exist anywhere but in hospitals—can cause infections. Now, not that you're anywhere near ready for Medicare, but it's worthy to note that this federal health plan for older Americans has taken the stance that so many hospital-acquired infections (called nosocomial infections in medical lingo) are preventable, so it will no longer pay hospitals and doctors for care needed to treat them!

Oh, Baby!

The risk for post-operative infection is so high that nearly all obstetricians in the United States routinely prescribe prophylactic antibiotic therapy following c-section and sometimes episiotomy.

If hospital birth has a higher likelihood for both interventions and complications, how can you make sure to have the least chance for either? The most effective strategy is to avoid the intervention, which correspondingly reduces the likelihood of complications. And if you're considering natural birth, that's already at the top of your priority list. Minimizing intervention requires you to be on the alert even before your admission. Many doctors and nurse midwives have *standing orders* for women admitted to the hospital birthing unit. Typically, these instructions have to do with matters such as IVs, fetal monitoring, what the woman can have to eat or drink, induction protocols, use of Pitocin, administration of pain medications, and exams or procedures the provider wants done. Standing orders are always in place for all patients admitted under the provider's name; to override them, the doctor or nurse midwife must specifically give a new order.

> **Birthing Book** _____
>
> **Standing orders** are pre-written instructions from a doctor or midwife that allow or direct hospital staff to take certain actions for all of that practitioner's patients when they're admitted to a hospital.

When you're planning a natural birth in a hospital, it's crucial for you to have your provider write specific preadmission orders for you that honor your choices and preferences. This is something to discuss early in your relationship with your provider so you can be assured this will happen. Otherwise, hospital staff will follow the existing standing orders. Establishing written birthing preferences is one of the most effective ways to avoid this pitfall.

The "*Do* Something!" Syndrome

We're not always so good, in our culture, at relaxing and going with the flow. We're busy, active, and in-charge people—and we like to always be doing something. It's not enough simply to drive to work; we have to be on the phone or bundling errands to make the most of our time and effort. This mindset spills over into almost every aspect of life. Within this mindset, the medical approach to birth feels familiar: it's action-driven. But when you're not the one who'll be doing the driving, "doing something" is likely to take you where you do not want to go.

For more than 90 percent of women who enter the hospital for birthing, this action begins with *continuous electronic fetal monitoring (CEFM)*. For CEFM, a nurse places two transducers on your belly, each held in place by a strap that goes around you. Cords run from the transducers to the display monitor. One transducer sends signals of your uterus's contractions, and the other sends signals of your baby's heartbeat.

> **Birthing Book** _____
>
> **Continuous electronic fetal monitoring (CEFM)** is an ultrasound technology that transmits, displays, and records signals of uterine contractions and the baby's heart rate.

CEFM debuted in the medical birth model in the 1970s, about the same time c-section became a standard obstetrical offering. The premise, then, was that monitoring the baby's heart rate could sound the alert when the baby was experiencing distress so that doctors could perform c-sections to save babies who otherwise wouldn't survive. CEFM has certainly led to more decisions to *do* c-sections—one third of women who have CEFM undergo what later turn out to be unnecessary c-sections. But there's no evidence to support CEFM as a lifesaving technology in routine, normal births. Life-threatening crises that arise out of nowhere are very uncommon.

It turns out all those beeps and jiggly lines on the monitor say very little about the baby's well-being in the end. Several well-done studies tell us that continuous electronic fetal monitoring does not change the outcome for the baby—that they don't save any babies in routine births because of this monitoring.

Fluctuations in the baby's heart rate and in the power and rate of contractions are normal and vary widely among women, but seeing (or hearing) every blip causes anxiety for moms as well as providers. Parents and staff alike huddle around the CEFM monitor. One little drop in the baby's heart rate—a variation that is likely normal—can create a sense of emergency in the parents. What good is it to be at the hospital if no one's going to *do* anything? It does become a compelling question after a while—why, exactly, is there all of this monitoring if it results in no benefit?

The entire setup becomes a lose-lose situation. Even studies of the reasons for CEFM note that the most common use of this technology is to defend malpractice lawsuits in court. Further, the monitor reinforces the idea that the mom should be in bed. Those cords, along with the IV and the blood pressure cuff, pretty much tether a woman in place. Then, there's no argument about getting up to walk around, take a shower, or even pee—which a woman should do every 60 to 90 minutes, but if she can't move around, well, there's *another* tube.

Having a nurse come in on a regular basis and use a handheld *fetal Doppler* (the same device your midwife or doctor uses to detect the baby's heartbeat during a prenatal visit) or a *fetoscope* is just as accurate at letting everyone know whether the baby needs help (or, most often, confirming that the baby is just fine). Doppler assessment means a nurse has to come into your room instead of being able to view a remote monitor at the nurse's station or rely on the system's preset warning levels to raise the alert when readings change.

> **Birthing Book** _____
>
> A **fetal Doppler** is a device that uses ultrasound to detect the baby's heart tones while the baby is in the uterus. The device then amplifies the tones and projects them as audible sounds. A **fetoscope** is a special stethoscope a practitioner uses to listen to the baby's heart (a method called auscultation). A fetoscope has a platform that braces against the practitioner's head to use bone conduction to amplify the heart sounds the stethoscope picks up.

Making the request for Doppler assessment may result in the nurse telling you the unit isn't really staffed to have a nurse keep running into your room to check on you all the time. So, the line of logic goes, it would be to your benefit to go with CEFM because then the technology will sound the alarm at the nurse's station of any irregularities, and—this is the part that's supposed to appease your concerns—keep staff intrusions to a minimum. Well, only you can decide whether this is a worthy trade-off. If you do choose to go with CEFM, turn the volume down or off in your room.

> **Trusty Midwife Tips** _____
>
> Hospitals approach CEFM, IVs, blood pressure monitoring, and even bladder catheterization as policies they enforce rather than options you can choose. Make sure you know early in your planning process, if you're intending to birth in a hospital, what the hospital's specific policies are. If you have no say—and especially if your provider also has no flexibility—choose a different hospital, a birthing center, or homebirth with a skilled midwife.

Genuine Danger or Scare Tactic?

It's sad but true that much of the practice of medicine today—not just with birthing—includes preventive measures (aka interventions) that are meant to cover providers when they have to defend their decisions and actions in court. Such measures are so common that they've become the standard.

When you fail to follow the routine by questioning the announced measures of care (because they're not presented to you as proposals or options)—or even flat-out refusing them—the tension ratchets up considerably. Sometimes, rather than simply answering your questions or asking you what your reasons are for refusing, doctors and hospital staff turn stern. "Do you really want to jeopardize your baby's well-being, not to mention your own?"

Of course you don't. The more you know, the more comfortable you can feel saying no—and also saying yes. You'll be confident that you've acquired enough knowledge yourself, and you've chosen providers you trust, to know when the circumstances clearly warrant the proposed intervention.

The Importance of Knowing Normal

Technology has its place and is certainly amazing when you genuinely need what it offers. However, it has become increasingly common for hospital staff and doctors to rely on technology to the near-exclusion of hands-on skills and experience. Few obstetricians or nurse midwives, for example, have ever assisted with a breech vaginal birth, so the approach to breech presentation is often c-section. But breech babies are among the natural variations in birth. Can they be problematic? Sure. Are they *inherently* problematic? No, only less common; about 10 percent of babies stay in a heads-up position when it comes time for birth. Genuine problems with birthing are fairly uncommon, but there are some situations that warrant further discussion because they can affect your birth: preeclampsia/eclampsia and placental abnormalities.

> **Oh, Baby!**
>
> Ask your practitioner to show you a sample *completed* informed consent document for a cesarean section. We emphasize the "completed" part because the surgeon has to write in the specific procedure and related risks. You'll be astonished.

Pressure's Rising

Preeclampsia is a funny word, although it sounds better than the old-fashioned term "toxemia of pregnancy." The word comes from ancient Greek words that mean "sudden out flash," probably referring to the sudden appearance of seizures. About 7 in 100 pregnant women develop preeclampsia, which is a condition that only occurs in humans during pregnancy. Its major signs are high blood pressure (hypertension) and protein in the urine (proteinuria). Fewer than 1 in 100 women who have preeclampsia go on to develop *eclampsia*, a life-threatening set of circumstances involving multiple body systems, internal fluid accumulation (edema), and seizures.

> **Birthing Book**
>
> **Preeclampsia** is a condition of pregnancy in which a woman develops high blood pressure and excess protein in the urine. **Eclampsia** is a life-threatening advancement of preeclampsia.

No one—not doctors, not researchers—knows how or why these conditions develop; accordingly, there aren't any clear ways to prevent them. There's some evidence that diet may be a significant factor; Chapter 9 takes a look at this topic. The current theory is that the sequence of events begins with an immune response to the placenta's implantation that results in inflammation affecting the lining of the blood vessels and organs, such as the kidneys. Although the baby's birth has long been the pivotal event in reversing the condition, researchers now believe it's actually the passing of the placenta that allows the mother's system to finally return to normal.

Because the deterioration of preeclampsia can lead to death, and preeclampsia never presents in the same fashion, any sign in the third trimester that could lead to preeclampsia should be investigated. Many women have swelling in the third trimester, protein in their urine, and an increase in blood pressure—the classic signs of preeclampsia. But these signs don't necessarily mean it *is* preeclampsia. They may simply be the typical third trimester discomforts and normal reaction to carrying an extra 35 pounds on the front of the body. However, for safety's sake more information must be gathered.

Blood tests give this information. Then everyone can relax or act with appropriate intervention. But if the condition worsens, the discussion about hastening birth will become more focused and intense. Because preeclampsia is most likely to develop later in pregnancy (32 weeks or beyond), induction or c-section becomes a very real possibility. The decision for an early birth (before 38 weeks) sets in motion a further set of interventions to help prepare the baby for life outside the womb, including medications to bring the baby's lungs to maturity. (Chapter 20 discusses these matters in detail.)

The Incredible Placenta

Abnormalities involving the placenta are among the most common, valid reasons for c-section. Fortunately, they're relatively *un*common—occurring in fewer than 1 in 100 pregnancies. The placenta is your baby's lifeline, so anything that compromises its ability to function is a threat to your baby's well-being. It also can be a threat to your well-being. The placenta is a blood organ, adhered to your uterus through thousands of tiny blood vessels. There are three placenta problems that may bring mention of risk and c-section:

◆ In **placenta accreta,** the placenta grows too deeply into the wall of the uterus, increasing the risk for difficulty separating after birth and the potential for excessive blood loss. Doctors typically detect placenta accreta with ultrasound done for another purpose; otherwise, there's no indication of it until after the birth, when the placenta does not detach. Many obstetricians prefer to schedule a surgical birth for women with detected placenta accreta. However, for many women it's perfectly fine to wait until after the birth; even if the placenta does not detach, manual removal is often sufficient and avoids a surgery.

◆ In **placenta previa,** the placenta grows so low in the uterus that it is near (marginal), encroaches on (moderate), or blocks (complete) the entrance to the birth path. The risk for uncontrolled bleeding with a vaginal birth is high when a woman has moderate placenta previa and nearly certain when she has complete placenta previa. Placenta previa is a medical situation that requires an obstetrician's care and, depending on how extensive, often a cesarean birth.

◆ **Placenta abruptio** occurs when the placenta detaches from the wall of the uterus before birth. It can be a medical emergency that requires an obstetrician's evaluation. A mild placenta abruptio can heal itself so the pregnancy can continue on its natural course. A significant placenta abruptio may require emergency intervention, including c-section, even when it means birthing the baby prematurely.

Do placental problems put the nix on a natural birth? Not necessarily. Mild placental abnormalities often don't affect the pregnancy and birth at all. Women who opt for a completely noninterventionary experience may not even know their placentas are anything other than normal. Factors that up the ante as far as risk, however, include preeclampsia and a previous c-section.

Scars on the wall of the uterus, no matter how well healed, alter the way the tissue can behave. Scar tissue is not as flexible as regular tissue and does not have the same blood supply. A placenta attached over the old c-section scar may not completely detach after the birth, causing a hemorrhage. The solution is to have an ultrasound scan in the third trimester to be sure that the placenta is not over the incision.

Some abnormalities actually aren't abnormal but have more to do with the timing of the ultrasound that detects them. A low-lying placenta is often picked up with an early ultrasound, leaving the parents very worried about the location of the placenta. But as the uterus grows, the placenta migrates—often moving away from the cervical opening (called the os). To see how this works, try this simple experiment: on a deflated balloon, draw a black dot about the size of a dime. Then blow up the balloon. See how the dot moves up the side of the balloon? It may even move all the way to the top. This is exactly what your placenta will do as your uterus grows.

Focus on What Matters

Sometimes people so entrench themselves in arguing their beliefs and positions and become so insistent on being right that they lose sight of what really matters: the best possible outcome for both the mother and baby. Statistics are great for being able to present a quantifiable picture that's bigger than your own (and your provider's) experience, but it's easy to get so wrapped up in the numbers that we forget to come back to what matters most: you and your individual, unique birth experience. Ten little fingers, ten little toes, two bright eyes, one tiny nose … these are the numbers that really matter, right?

The Least You Need to Know

- There is no evidence to support the perspective that natural birth in any environment, including the home, is unsafe in a normal, routine pregnancy.

- The most frequent reason women of child-bearing age are hospitalized is to give birth.

- Infection is a very real concern when you're hospitalized; the germ population of a hospital is extensive and often unfamiliar to your immune system, making you more vulnerable.

- Even when there are problems in pregnancy that could pose risks during birth, there are often noninterventionary methods for dealing with them.

Chapter 7

Making a Choice: Midwife or Doctor?

In This Chapter

◆ To get what you want, you have to shop around

◆ So many players, so many possibilities

◆ Midwives are not all the same

◆ Doctors occupy the spectrum from holistic to specialist

◆ Interviewing prospective providers

You can talk a good game when it comes to what you'd like your birth experience to be, but what are you doing to make sure you can play it the way you're planning it? You have to put in place the proper team to help you make it happen, yet most women do less comparison shopping for a birth-care provider than for groceries!

Who you choose as your provider for care during pregnancy and birth is a pivotal decision when you want to have a natural birth. You have to choose someone you trust to give you honest information and help you make decisions that keep you on track with the birth you envision—and someone who respects and trusts you. And, of course, you need someone who has all the right stuff when it comes to qualifications and skills.

Shop Around

You have specific and unique expectations. A provider's clinical expertise and experience might be just the ticket for meeting them, but when the two of you meet, it could be like trying to align the wrong ends of magnets. Providers don't get along with everyone for all kinds of reasons; they don't expect you to, either. It's okay to shop around for a midwife or doctor. In fact, most expect and encourage it—it's the only way to find the best match.

It seems a natural birth would be an option in every provider's repertoire. But sadly, as you may have already discovered, this is not the case. Even more distressing is that you often must ferret out those who say they support natural birth but really don't or so broadly define natural birth that it covers anything short of a c-section (not!). Some providers (most often doctors, but sometimes midwives, too) will even agree with everything you say and want but secretly believe you'll end up doing things their way because they're the experts. This usually turns out to be the case, because the ship sails where the captain says.

> **Trusty Midwife Tips**
>
> Other women who have recently birthed are often your best filter for separating the hype from the practice. Most women are eager to talk to you about their experiences with a midwife or doctor. A doctor's nurse is often a good source of information, too. You'll be amazed what you can find out simply through ordinary conversation.

If a provider is known for "always" performing an episiotomy or for doing c-sections to "avoid" problems, what can you do to be sure you would be an exception—and more importantly, what makes you believe you *can* be an exception? Philosophical differences seldom resolve themselves in ways that make both sides happy. Later in this chapter, we give you the 20 questions that'll help you cut to the core in terms of expressing your own views as well as defining those of the provider.

If you do settle on a provider and then later discover that the two of you have fundamental differences in your beliefs about the birthing process, change providers. Those differences won't change, and it's not going to be your philosophy that comes out on top. The provider would prefer you find someone who is on the same page with you, too. No one wants to enter a relationship knowing from the start that it's going to be contentious.

Getting Down to Your Short List

Open the Yellow Pages and you're certain to find an overwhelming selection of doctors, midwives, and birthing services and facilities. (Chapter 8 talks about birthing places.) You could close your eyes and plant your finger. Or you could start by asking women who have young kids who they went to and what they thought of their experiences. Could you ask your primary care provider for recommendations, too? Well, sure you could … but never underestimate the power of women's direct experiences. We encourage you to take advantage of social networks to gather as much firsthand information as you can!

Friends and family members are an easy place to start, and for some you may have been involved in some way with their birthing experiences—so you'll have some first-hand perceptions to add to the mix. You see moms with their babies everywhere—ask them, too, even if you don't know who they are. Just be general and friendly. Most mothers are eager to say something about their providers. You'll get more than enough information to whittle down that list to a manageable few.

Pick six or so providers that seem promising and call their offices to schedule interview appointments. Many providers offer interview appointments at no charge. Some may not be taking new clients, so be prepared for that. At your interview, ask each provider the same questions, and write down the answers so you can then go home and compare. (We give you a list of suggested questions later in this chapter.)

Go Together

Take your baby's father, your partner, your sister, your friend, your mom—whoever you may intend to be part of the birthing experience. At the very least, take along someone whose opinion you trust. With another person there, you'll get another perspective. If it's the same as yours, great. And if you love the provider but the other person says, "I couldn't wait to get out of there!", then you have a lively conversation for the trip home to figure out why.

It's often helpful to have another set of eyes, ears, and observations. You may connect—or not—with a particular provider for reasons that blind you to concerns you should have. Sometimes even though two people hear the same response, each hears something different. We all have our own set of filters for processing information. Try to have the person who goes with you to the interview appointment write down the provider's responses, too, so you can compare your perceptions.

Who's Who ... The Major Players

Lots of folks are lined up out there just waiting for your business. Each has something unique to offer; your task is to find the one who has what you want. This isn't as easy a task as it might sound, though, because some of the players aren't quite what they seem or you expect. Just because a provider is a midwife doesn't mean she supports natural birth, nor do all doctors haul out the big bag of interventions as soon as you walk through the door. Credentials are essential, but they don't define the provider's abilities or philosophy. You have to search, investigate, and choose with care.

Who's Who in Birthing

Obstetrician	Physician; surgical specialist; often considered "the best"; rarely sees a normal, low-risk birth during many years of specialized training
Family practitioner	Physician; primary care provider; holistic approach to health, medicine, and birth; usually will provide care for pregnant women and attend births (although not all do)
General practitioner	Physician; primary care provider; holistic approach to health and medicine; may or may not take pregnant clients and attend births; this type of provider is increasingly rare (you are more likely to find family practitioners today)
Physician assistant	Exactly what it says; in rural areas may be the only primary care provider available; may be independently practicing; has a greater scope of practice than a nurse practitioner (but they most often do not do prenatal care or births)
Nurse practitioner	Registered nurse; able to provide a broad range of health-care services; may be independently practicing
Certified nurse midwife	A registered nurse who takes additional training for attending births; most often found in the hospital setting or a hospital birthing center; must have physician back-up; bound by hospital policy (some do homebirths and birth center births)
Certified midwife	Independent midwife with national professional licensing; all formal, supervised education and training relate to normal, low-risk birth; not a nurse; follows evidence-based policies and protocols

Direct-entry midwife	Independent midwife with a state license; all formal, supervised education and training relate to normal, low-risk birth; not a nurse; follows evidence-based policies and protocols; may do homebirths and births in independent birthing centers
Licensed midwife	Usually a catch-all description for either a certified professional midwife or a direct-entry midwife who has a state license
Lay midwife	Independent midwife who receives her training through experience and observation; not a nurse; not acknowledged or recognized by the medical model
Doula	Labor and birth supporter; advocates on behalf of the birthing woman; not a health-care provider

Midwives

Lots of women will tell you that they had a midwife for their birth, but what kind of midwife did they have? There is a big difference between a nurse midwife who usually works in the hospital and a homebirth midwife who attends your birth at home.

Overall, midwives offer the least intrusive, most supportive birthing experience, so many women planning or considering a natural birth look to midwives for their pregnancy care and birthing assistance. Although midwives in general offer a more holistic and integrated approach, their philosophies and practice styles are by no means the same. What kind of midwife is available to you depends on where you live; state laws determine credentialing, licensing, and other requirements that define what midwives can do.

In the United States, there are two kinds of midwives: *nurse midwives* and *direct-entry midwives*. There is about the same number of each—roughly 4,000—currently in practice. Combined, midwives assist at about 8 percent of births in the United States, unlike in Europe where midwives assist at more than 75 percent of births.

Most nurse midwives assist at births in birthing centers and hospitals; they are usually not autonomous practitioners and seldom do homebirths. Nurse midwives work under the direct guidance of physicians. Direct-entry midwives assist at homebirths and births in free-standing birthing centers that are not affiliated with hospitals (more about this in Chapter 8); they seldom assist with hospital-based births, although they may be present at the mom's request to act as advocate and *doula*.

Homebirth midwives are completely autonomous practitioners and are experts in normal birth. If they are licensed by the state they live in or if they hold a national license, they have guidelines and protocols as well. Midwifery protocols are written from evidence-based data about birth. Most homebirth midwives have hospital backup and a strong relationship with a homebirth-friendly doctor they can talk to about anything that's outside the convention of low risk or normal.

> **Birthing Book** _____
>
> **Nurse midwives** are registered nurses (RNs) who have additional education and certification in midwifery. **Direct-entry midwives** have specific training and experience in birthing and may be certified and/or licensed but are not nurses. A **doula** is a birth assistant who provides labor support such as personal care, comfort, and advocacy during the birthing process but does not become directly involved in the birth. A **lay midwife** acquires her expertise through experience and assists with homebirths.

A *lay midwife* has training based primarily in experience and observation. Lay midwives exclusively assist at homebirths or births in nonhospital birthing centers.

Certified Nurse Midwife (CNM)

A nurse midwife is a registered nurse (RN) who completes additional education and training and passes a certification test to earn the designation Certified Nurse Midwife (CNM). However, in some states midwifery is an area of nursing specialization within licensing and certification as an Advanced Registered Nurse Practitioner (ARNP). Nurse midwives have one foot in the medical model and one foot in the midwifery model, although when push comes to shove they are medical practitioners by both training and licensure. If you want a natural birth but will be birthing in a hospital or a hospital-affiliated birthing center, a nurse midwife is your best chance for making that happen.

A nurse midwife might see a dozen or more women and assist with as many births in a week and may have thousands of births under her belt. She may refer to you as a patient or a client depending on where she has positioned herself along the medical-midwifery spectrum. Your prenatal appointments with a nurse midwife may last 20 to 30 minutes, so you have plenty of opportunity to ask questions and discuss how you're feeling. These visits generally are more casual and relaxed than the ones you'd have with a doctor, and by the time of your birth the nurse midwife will know your family, your interests, and probably the names of your pets.

Although most nurse midwives support natural birth, their training and licensing as RNs gives them the ability to quickly step across the line to start an IV, administer medications, or do an episiotomy. In nearly all states, nurse midwives are permitted to practice only in association with a physician. The physician establishes the guidelines within which the nurse midwife can act. The structure is one of teamwork; the nurse midwife is part of the medical team that the doctor leads. Nurse midwives may also provide routine women's health services such as annual exams and Pap smears.

Direct-Entry Midwife

Direct-entry midwives are not nurses. Many receive their training through the "each one teach one" apprenticeship or preceptor model, which combines formal education (as a blend of college, workshops, and other training) with practical experience. They may choose to earn the Certified Professional Midwife (CPM) national credential through the North American Registry of Midwives (NARM), although they are not required to do so. Direct-entry midwives are really the core of the midwifery model and offer the best circumstance for natural birth at home or in a midwife-directed birthing center. They may also choose to become licensed midwives, depending on the state in which they practice.

Direct-entry midwives and CPMs have formal training in normal birth, which they attain in several different ways. "Direct entry" means that the midwife learned directly by attending births and took a specified training course and now has a certificate or license. Such a training course may be on-site at a birthing facility, through a midwifery college, or through didactic modules via the Internet. Regardless, all avenues of direct-entry midwifery training further require hands-on training with direct supervision.

It takes at least two years to accomplish all the necessary book learning and hands-on training needed to pass the certifying or licensing test—all of which is about pregnancy, birth, postpartum, newborns, breastfeeding, CPR, and neonatal resuscitation (and in some states, starting IVs, administering IV fluids, and carrying birth-related medications). On top of this, most direct-entry midwives have training in multiple complementary medicine techniques such as herbal remedies or massage.

Most states require some sort of licensing for direct-entry midwives, although qualifications and criteria vary widely. Direct-entry midwives are not required to have structured, formal working relationships with physicians, although most have informal and strong relationships with local doctors who support natural birth and to whom the midwife can turn when a medical situation arises. A few states directly outlaw direct-entry midwives or have laws that are so restrictive that there's little practical difference.

You can expect a direct-entry midwife to refer to you as a client (or simply by name). She might see 8 to 10 women a month and has assisted at several dozen to perhaps hundreds of births over her career, depending on how long she has been a midwife. A direct-entry midwife plans to be with you for the duration of your birthing process and gives you as much time as you desire during your visits before the birth. Direct-entry midwives generally integrate a wide range of complementary practices and therapies, ranging from herbal teas and meditation methods to hypnosis and water-birth. (Later chapters discuss these approaches and more.) Certified Professional Midwives (CPMs) also may provide routine health exams for women.

> **Trusty Midwife Tips** _____
>
> Want to find the status of midwifery in your state? The Citizens for Midwifery website provides a state-by-state guide. Visit the website at cfmidwifery.org/states. The Midwives Alliance of North America (MANA) also maintains information about legal issues related to midwifery. MANA's website is mana.org/statechart.html.

Lay Midwife

Lay midwives learn what they know through assisting at births rather than through formal education. They are the fewest in number among midwives, and because they're not licensed or certified, it's hard to know how many are actually out there. Some of them make it a point to fly under the radar, tending to birthing women only through word of mouth. It can be more difficult to objectively evaluate a lay midwife's qualifications; references are especially important.

Doulas

Although not actually health-care providers, doulas float the most freely between the medical and midwifery models in the services they provide for birthing women. You might think of a doula as your labor support person—she does everything from fixing you hot tea and helping you in and out of the birthing tub to calming your birthing partner and ever so firmly telling the nurses that yes, you are indeed certain you do not want an epidural, as well as helping you through each and every contraction.

The classic interpretation of the word doula is "with woman," but if you look up the Greek definition of doula, you'll find that it means "servant." This is not too far from the truth; a doula supports and serves the laboring woman and family. Most will see you once or twice prenatally, will attend your birth, and will visit once or twice after the birth. Some will offer to labor with you at home before you go to the hospital; some will just meet you at the hospital.

Doulas are occasionally hospital employees, which somewhat restricts their roles because they have to follow hospital policies and procedures. This may mean a doula could reach the line where she can no longer advocate for your preferences when they clash with hospital protocols. On the flip side, a hospital doula can be an advantage for you because she knows the ins and outs of the hospital experience and can help you work the system to your benefit. Most doulas are independent, however. You may hire a doula through your midwife or find one on your own. Having an independent doula at your birth provides the most options for you.

> **Trusty Midwife Tips**
>
> A midwife may sometimes serve as a doula—for example, if you've started out at home with a midwife and then find that you need the care of a physician. However, a doula is not a midwife and never serves in that function!

Some doulas are certified; some are not. Some doulas work from a base of experience without having had any formal training. Others complete a three-day workshop of training to learn the most effective ways to interact with the medical model yet advocate for the mom. A doula's sole agenda is to help you have your best birth. Chapter 16 is all about doulas.

Physicians

Doctors are the big kahunas of the birthing business; they attend 92 percent of births in the United States. Pretty much all of those births take place in a hospital or hospital-affiliated birthing center. The doctor who assists with a homebirth is rarer a breed among physicians than one who makes house calls. As you remember from earlier chapters, the medical profession worked very hard to move birth from the home to the hospital, and doctors today are fairly well indoctrinated for hospital birth; they are the embodiment of the medical model for birthing.

Physicians who provide care for pregnancy and birth may be MDs (doctor of medicine) or DOs (doctor of osteopathy). They typically specialize in family medicine or in obstetrics. Although family medicine is broad-based, what many people think of as general practice is a *board-certified specialty*. Obstetrics is also a board-certified specialty. Obstetricians provide care only during pregnancy, birth, and the few weeks following birth. Many obstetricians are also gynecologists, providing a full spectrum of medical care for women outside the sphere of pregnancy.

> **Birthing Book**
>
> A **board-certified specialty** is an area of medical practice that requires several years of focused training, after which the physician must pass written, oral, and skills examinations to receive board certification. A **physician assistant (PA)** is a medical practitioner who provides basic to mid-level medical care under the authority of a physician.

A doctor may also have a *physician assistant (PA)* who provides complete care for normal, routine pregnancies and births. A PA follows a course of education and training very similar to that of an MD but about two years shorter and without a three- to four-year residency to become board-certified. PAs may specialize in many of the same fields as doctors and receive certification in their specialties just as physicians do. In most states, PAs can prescribe medications, diagnose and treat medical conditions, perform minor surgeries and procedures, and assist at major surgeries. If you go to a PA for your pregnancy and birth, you'll have pretty much the same experience as if you go to a doctor.

Surgical Specialist: The Obstetrician

Obstetricians are specialists in identifying and fixing what goes wrong during pregnancy and birth. Some truly focus on the specialist end of things, caring for women whose pregnancies are high risk—women carrying higher multiples (triplets or more), women who have conceived through fertility treatments, women who have serious underlying health conditions, or women who develop medical problems during pregnancy.

Because only 20 percent (or less) of pregnancies truly need such a high level of medical attention, most obstetricians also provide care for women whose pregnancies are normal and routine. This is especially true in urban areas, where obstetricians provide 90 percent or more of the care for pregnancy and birth. There's also the philosophical slant that providing routine care in normal situations improves the specialist's ability to detect and treat problems and difficulties.

Some obstetricians are very supportive of natural birth and are very good at coaching women through the birthing process without unnecessary interventions. Your best chance to find one of them is to look for those who promote and provide *integrative care*. But ultimately, obstetrics is a surgical specialty, and what a surgeon knows and does best is surgery. Obstetricians have the highest rate of birthing interventions. Not that this is either bad or negative; indeed, in the right circumstances, an obstetrician is the ideal choice when it's what you need for the best outcome.

> **Birthing Book**
>
> **Integrative care** is an approach that blends conventional (often called allopathic) medicine with other therapeutic methods such as acupuncture, herbal therapies, and meditation.

If you want to receive your care from an obstetrician in a hospital with a medical model mindset but you want a natural birth, you'll likely need to advocate for it—sometimes strongly and every step of the way. You also need to realize and accept that you may not be able to shake the paradigm enough to get the natural birth experience you want. Think about going to a Volkswagen dealership to buy a Mercedes. You may actually get a Mercedes if the dealership has enough pull to get one in for you. But most likely, you're going to drive away in a Volkswagen.

Obstetricians share call responsibilities with other obstetricians in the area, either within their own practice groups or collectively across several practices. Your OB may or may not be on call when you arrive at the hospital. Very rarely will an obstetrician come in for a birth when it's not his or her night to be on call. The odds that your own obstetrician will be present for your birth could be one in seven or even less if the call roster is large enough.

The potential dilemma for you is that if you've worked hard to negotiate an understanding with your obstetrician about your birth experience, you could find yourself in the care of a different obstetrician who disagrees. Chapter 17 talks about how to make a birthing preferences plan that makes your desires and agreements clear for any practitioner who might step into your care picture.

Emphasis on the Bigger Picture: The Family Practitioner

The farther you live from a major city, the more likely you'll find family practitioners who provide care during pregnancy and assist at birthing. Family practitioners spend part of their specialty training in care for women during pregnancy and birth. But fewer than half, overall, end up offering such care when they enter practice—and in urban areas where obstetricians have the corner on the birthing market, it may be next to impossible to find a family practitioner who does births.

A family practitioner is more holistic than an obstetrician by training and by philosophy. The family practitioner looks not only at the person who is the patient but also considers the family and community setting as a whole, along with emotional, social, environmental, and other facets of everyday life that influence both health and disease. If you want to receive care during pregnancy and birth from a doctor and yet still have a natural birth, a family practitioner is your best bet.

Family practitioners are in short supply and very busy, though, and many take only a certain number of maternity patients. Partly, this is because there's such unpredictability to birth—babies come when they want to, not because it's two o'clock on a Tuesday afternoon and there just happens to be space in the doctor's schedule to dash to the hospital.

Oh, Baby!

Although a typical prenatal visit with a doctor may be scheduled for 20 minutes, studies show that you'll get 6 to 10 minutes with the doctor. The rest of the visit is about health measures (such as weight and blood pressure), lab tests, and other things the nurse or medical assistant handles.

Your typical visit with a family practitioner is likely to be about 10 minutes. However, in a busy practice you may see a physician assistant or a nurse practitioner as well (or instead), so overall you may spend 20 minutes with someone during your routine appointments. The family practitioner may take a call himself or herself and at least be in contact with the hospital when you arrive, but is likely to come to check on you rather than stay at the hospital. Most family practitioners want to be present at the birth, although some follow an on-call schedule for after-hours births that may result in another doctor in the practice group being the one who's there for your birth.

Trusty Midwife Tips

Whatever happened to the trusty GP, the good doctor who did a little of everything? Well, he or she has pretty much fallen by the wayside in our current paradigm of specialization, replaced by the family practitioner—a specialist in family medicine. Some American doctors still do complete medical school and internship and then decide to enter general practice. GPs are increasingly fewer in number in the United States.

Twenty Questions: Interviewing Your Provider-to-Be

You wouldn't take a job just because there was an ad in the paper. You'd expect to at least have an interview. During the interview, you may discover the job's not what you thought it would be, that you don't much like the people or the work environment, or that the hours don't suit your needs. And you wouldn't hesitate to turn down the job—politely, of course. Nor would you, if you were a business owner or supervisor, hire someone who called about a job without first interviewing him or her. You'd want to make sure the person is qualified for the job and seems like a good fit with the energy and purpose of the business you do, even if all that means is that you think you could get along with this person, day in and day out.

So why would you approach choosing a health-care provider any differently? When you're choosing a provider, you're hiring someone with the right credentials, experience, and mindset to match your needs and expectations. You're also establishing a fairly long-term relationship in which mutual trust and respect are essential. So get out your pen ... you have work to do!

Interview Questions for Your Provider-to-Be

The answers to these 20 questions will give you a good framework for comparing providers to choose the one who most closely matches the kind of birth experience you want to have. You may have other questions to add to the list; just make sure to ask the same questions of each provider. We've put some lines for you to write down the answers; you can photocopy these pages and take them along with you on your interview appointments.

1. How long have you been in practice, and how many births do you assist in a year or over the course of your practice?

   _____

   _____

2. I want a natural birth. What does that mean to you, and how do you feel about natural birth? How would you go about helping me achieve a natural birth?

   _____

   _____

3. How many births that you assist happen in a hospital?

   _____

   _____

4. How many births that you assist happen in a birthing center?

_____

_____

5. How many births that you assist are homebirths? Of those homebirths, how many end up as transports to the hospital?

_____

_____

6. What are the circumstances in which you might induce or augment labor?

_____

_____

7. How do you determine whether labor is progressing?

_____

_____

8. Is there an amount of time for a woman to be in labor that you're generally comfortable with as normal, after which you begin considering interventions? If so, what are those interventions?

_____

_____

9. At how many births that you assist does the woman get an epidural? An episiotomy?

_____

_____

10. At how many births do you use assistive methods such as forceps or vacuum extraction? What are your criteria for making the decision?

_____

_____

11. How many births that you assist are c-sections? What are your criteria for determining that a c-section is necessary?

    _____

    _____

12. Are there situations in which you always do a c-section?

    _____

    _____

13. What complementary methods for my comfort and relaxation during the birth process do you encourage or support? Besides drugs, how do you help mothers stay as comfortable as possible throughout their labors?

    _____

    _____

14. What do you know about hypnosis for comfort during birthing?

    _____

    _____

15. What do you know about waterbirth?

    _____

    _____

16. Can I be in the position that's most comfortable and effective for me when I birth my baby?

    _____

    _____

17. Who may be present for, and participate in, the birth?

    _____

    _____

18. Does my baby stay with me following birth? Will a nurse take my baby away from me to be weighed and examined? Can I request bedside exams?

_____

_____

19. Will you be with me for my birth? If not, who will be?

_____

_____

20. How do you help mothers with breastfeeding?

_____

_____

You might have other questions specific to your unique circumstances, too. Among these might be:

◆ If you have diabetes, high blood pressure, or other ongoing health conditions that are being successfully treated: Can you have a natural birth?

◆ How do your options change, in the provider's perspective, if you have genital herpes, hepatitis B, or group-B strep?

◆ How do your options change if it turns out you're carrying multiples?

Of course, you'll have lots and lots of questions over the course of your pregnancy. But the answers to these questions will help you choose the provider who you'll be most comfortable with for your care—and who you'll trust to answer all those other questions.

Making Sense of the Answers

It's a good idea to go through these questions yourself first and write the answers that you'd find most supportive of your interests. With a natural birth as your goal, you're looking for the least intervention; so keep in mind that the answers you get will be different depending on the kind of provider you're interviewing.

An obstetrician is likely to have a high rate of c-sections and episiotomies, for example, and it'll be hard for you to determine whether this is because he or she cares for a lot of medically complicated births or has care guidelines that favor early intervention. A direct-entry midwife, on the other hand, may have no episiotomies and only one birth in a year that ends in c-section.

The Least You Need to Know

♦ One of the most important decisions you'll make about your birth is choosing your provider; your provider greatly affects the kind of birthing experience you can have.

♦ Providers define natural birth in as many different ways as anyone else; it's crucial to make sure you and your provider share the same definition.

♦ Family practitioners are generally the most holistic among physicians; obstetricians are the most specialized and by training are surgery-oriented.

♦ The philosophies and scopes of practice of the different kinds of midwives vary widely; just because she's a midwife doesn't mean she's a match for you and the birth experience you desire.

♦ It's important to interview and compare different providers; ask the same questions of each, and write down the answers so when you go back home you can objectively evaluate the information you've gathered.

Chapter 8

Homebirth, Birthing Center, or Hospital?

In This Chapter

- ◆ All the comforts of home
- ◆ Choosing a birthing center
- ◆ The hospital birth
- ◆ The politics and business of birthing
- ◆ Making choices to get the birth experience you want

Location, location, location. This familiar mantra of the real estate agent holds a message for you, too. It's not that you need curb appeal—you have plenty of that going for you! Rather, the message is that you need to think about where you're going to have a natural birth so you can choose the place most likely to give you the birthing experience you desire.

The three most common settings—hospital, birthing center, and home—differ in crucial ways. You may think you already know what these differences mean and how they influence your plans and wishes. But do you?

The Right Place

You probably didn't think that much about where you'd birth your baby until you started exploring natural birth and the world of options flew wide open. A lot of people don't give a second thought to where they'll give birth. Many assume a hospital is the only place to go, and if they do think about where they're going to birth, they're busy trying to figure out the fastest way to get there. But where you choose to be for your birth is the second-most important decision (the first being your choice of provider) you need to make when you want a natural birth.

If you've been thinking about natural birth for a while, maybe you've been considering a birthing center, or maybe you're toying with the idea that you might not even want to *go* anywhere—you might want a homebirth. Keep in mind that your provider choice affects the birthing place you choose. Doctors (especially obstetricians), for example, seldom assist at births outside the hospital, although family practitioners do sometimes assist at births in birthing centers. On the other hand, direct-entry midwives don't assist births in hospitals.

Who Assists Where

Home	Birthing Center	Hospital
Direct-Entry Midwife (DEM);	Certified Nurse Midwife (CNM);	OB; FP; CNM
Certified Professional Midwife (CPM);	CPM; Family Practitioner (FP);	
Licensed Midwife (LM); Lay Midwife	Obstetrician (OB)	

Home Is Where the Heart Lives

You can read until your eyes fall out, and you can take childbirth classes until you could teach them yourself. Unless you're willing to take the reins of your own birth and decide what you want and what is best for you and your baby, though, anything else you do won't matter a bit. Homebirth puts you squarely in the driver's seat for your birthing experience.

Imagine being able to snack during your labor and putter around the house or be out in the yard until your labor demands more of your attention, letting your baby come on its own schedule, in its own time. Picture being in your own pajamas or wearing nothing but your birthday suit if that's what you prefer. Envision sharing this most intimate experience with your partner, in privacy and in comfort, with no worries about unexpected intrusions. In fact, you can have whoever you want with you at home; who is present with you as you give birth is totally up to you and will be different for different people.

See yourself in the shower or bathtub or taking any position you want at any time during your labor and feeling relaxed and trusting enough in your body that you can actually feel your baby descending and feel that your body is progressing. How good would it be to not be afraid of the power of your own body? How nice would it be for the baby to come right to your chest, moments after birth, and never leave your arms until you say so?

This is homebirth: birth in your own environment, with your own "stuff" and the people you love nearby—quietly talking, reading, playing cards, or even napping. Picture it: everyone is calm and relaxed, including you, waiting in happy anticipation to meet the new baby. You know what's happening in your body; you're in tune with the changes taking place. You feel your baby's preparations as the time approaches for your baby to leave your body and enter into life on its own. You're confident in your ability to do this, and your mind and body are synchronized and focused on creating the birth you want.

When you choose homebirth, you're free to move around, do yoga, eat, drink, sleep, stand in the shower, sit in the tub—whatever you want, when and how you want. You can be in any position that makes you most comfortable. You decide who you want to be there with you, and how you want to interact with them. Maybe you don't want to talk, or maybe you have a lot on your mind you'd like to share.

Sometimes homebirth can seem anticlimactic. When a woman feels safe and private, her hormones usually work exactly as they should, so labor usually progresses with efficiency. The birth is happening, and everyone is calm. When mom feels safe and private, the baby does, too.

> **Oh, Baby!**
>
> Homebirth is a great option for all the benefits it offers. However, if you're considering homebirth solely because you do not have medical insurance or the resources to pay for care, please contact a midwife in your area. Midwives are often able to negotiate ways to work with you so you can safely have the birthing experience you desire.

> **Natural Woman**
>
> Sometimes birth takes place spontaneously while you're waiting for the midwife to arrive (or, more notoriously, in the backseat of the car on the way to the birthing center or hospital). Most often, such a birth turns out just fine for both mom and baby—the baby is healthy and strong and apparently was just ready to enter the world.

Factors to Consider with a Homebirth

Some people worry about things such as the mess and the smell of birthing at home. Are you going to have to repaint the walls and get new furniture? Well, only if those renovations were on the agenda to start with! Birthing involves some fluid, most of it amniotic (not blood)—and not as much as it seems.

In a hospital, everything is designed to make cleanup as fast and easy as possible. Basins and towels catch most of the fluids, and the birthing woman doesn't really have any sense of what is going on beyond the sensations of her baby arriving—she's pretty preoccupied. Also, she's lying on a birthing bed or table designed to flow all the fluids and discharges right into those collection basins.

Hospitals are also obsessed—and rightfully so—with the fact that those fluids are your fluids, and they don't want them to touch anything else. It's a perspective, realistically, that you want them to have because you don't want someone else's "stuff" mingling with yours. There are all kinds of new germs at the hospital that could cause problems for you or your baby, so universal precautions are crucial.

But at home, it's *all* yours. Anything your baby could be exposed to is already familiar—from dog and cat hair to bird feathers to anything else living in your house (even germs). And most homebirth midwives are very aware of how things look and make every effort to keep things tidy and welcoming to anyone present for the birth.

At a homebirth, the midwife covers the bed and floor around it with absorbent, vinyl-backed pads to contain the fluids and quickly replaces them when they become saturated. You can also drape other furniture, such as your sofa or favorite chair, with waterproof covers and absorbent towels. There's not much cleaning left to do after the birth, and typically the midwife or doula takes care of it. You're left with a clean, comfortable home.

What About the Kids?

If you have other children at home, you'll need to make a decision about whether they should, or want to, be present for the birth. Factors to consider include the children's ages, interest in being part of the birth, and ability to listen and appropriately behave. Younger children especially may need such a level of attention from you that you feel drawn away from your birthing experience.

Some women choose to have other children present, though have another adult there who is responsible for overseeing them. You want your partner free to be there for you, so this should be someone else. Ideally, if you have other children you've involved them in some way in discussions about the birth so they know it is natural and normal, and so they have some idea what to expect.

Homebirth: The Politics and the Controversy

We'd be remiss if we failed to discuss the controversy that homebirth arouses. Both the American College of Obstetrics and Gynecology (ACOG) and the American Medical Association (AMA), professional organizations of physicians, have issued formal position statements opposing homebirth—assisted or unassisted—asserting unequivocally that:

> "...the safest setting for labor, delivery, and the immediate post-partum period is in the hospital, or a birthing center within a hospital complex, that meets standards jointly outlined by the American Academy of Pediatrics (AAP) and ACOG, or in a freestanding birthing center that meets the standards of the Accreditation Association for Ambulatory Health Care, the Joint Commission, or the American Association of Birth Centers."

> —ACOG press release, February 8, 2008

ACOG's position statement further criticizes that "lay or other midwives attending to homebirths are unable to perform lifesaving emergency cesarean deliveries and other surgical and medical procedures that would best safeguard the mother and child." True enough! Surgery and medical procedures are *clearly* the venue of the physician; no one challenges this point. Further, no one challenges that a hospital is the best place for such procedures. But in August 2008, the AMA voted to support the ACOG's position as well as its official call for federal legislation to make home-birth illegal throughout the United States.

Although these positions are ostensibly to support the safety, health, and well-being of women and newborns, the numbers fail to support them (see Chapter 6). They're positions that inherently remove choice and autonomy in birth—which even ACOG acknowledges is a natural process—from women. Such stridency does not exist in any other circumstance of health or health care or in any other country. The American College of Nurse-Midwives has issued a comparably unequivocal statement challenging the position of the ACOG and the AMA, noting that the physician group statements ignore data from reputable studies that show homebirth to be no more risky than hospital birth—not to mention much lower in medical intervention and its related complications.

Natural Woman

Former talk-show host Ricki Lake's 2007 documentary film, *The Business of Being Born,* appears to have fueled the home-birth debate as well as spurred a surge in women seeking birthing assistance from midwives. In the film, which showcases Lake's own homebirth, Lake takes a critical view of medical birth.

Birthing Centers

In most birthing centers, the birthing mom gets a suite that is at least a large enough room to walk around or set up a birthing tub if she wants to do so. There's space enough for her partner and others she has invited to the birth to settle in and be comfortable, too—often including at least one extra bed. Her support team can be available when she wants them, yet quietly unobtrusive when she wants to sleep or relax.

There's also usually a generous bathroom with a spacious shower and bathtub big enough for soaking. In larger birthing centers, birthing suites may have separate kitchens and additional rooms. The birthing mom can eat what she wants, when she wants, and can have music and soft lighting. Some birthing centers even allow incense and candles as long as local fire regulations permit them. Hmm … sounds more like an oceanfront retreat than home! But that's part of the intent: to provide a sense of cocooning so birthing moms can give full focus to the reason they're there: birthing.

Many birthing centers give a woman complete freedom to birth how she wants to, including waterbirth. Not all birthing centers allow waterbirth, though, so this is something to verify if you think you want one. (Chapter 14 is all about waterbirth.) Birthing center staff members are mostly Certified Nurse Midwives (CNMs), although some have Certified Professional Midwives (CPMs), too, as well as doulas and other support people. Medical insurance that pays for a hospital birth nearly always pays for a birthing center birth as long as the center is staffed with CNMs or is an extension of the hospital, but this is an important detail to verify with your insurance carrier as well as with the birthing center that you're considering.

There are about 180 birthing centers in the United States, many of which are owned and operated by nurse midwives and others by hospitals. What a particular birthing center can offer and how it operates varies among states because states set the licensing requirements. Birthing centers do not offer surgery, and most don't offer medications (except local anesthetic to suture tears). So they screen birthing moms carefully to make sure they're prepared for a natural birth. But if your provider is a midwife, you have already passed the screening because midwives assist only with normal, routine pregnancies and births.

Natural Woman

Because birthing centers do not offer surgery, there's no expectation that a birth "might" end up as a c-section. Instead, there's every expectation that birth will unfold exactly as designed. Studies show that among women who birth at birthing centers, about 5 percent have c-sections compared with the national rate of more than 32 percent.

Having your birth in a birthing center will be, of course, a more structured experience than birthing at home. Birthing centers have policies, protocols, and procedures they must follow to meet regulatory (laws) and insurance (malpractice) requirements. Time becomes a key measure of progress during labor, although there's generally much more latitude than in a hospital—as well as much less pressure for medical interventions (such as Pitocin to augment labor and electronic fetal monitoring)—because those are simply not available at the birthing center.

If any issues arise during birthing to require medical attention and intervention, the birthing center will transport you to a hospital for whatever treatment you need. Statistics show that about 35 percent of first-time moms and 10 percent of repeat moms end up being transferred from a birthing center to a hospital for birthing; about 5 percent overall have c-sections. About half of these transfers are at the woman's request rather than because of a medical emergency—for example, her pain is more than she can manage so she wants an epidural or other medication. Some women simply decide they would feel more comfortable surrounded by the latest technology.

The Midwifery Birthing Center

Most freestanding birthing centers in the United States are owned and operated by midwives (usually CNMs). Because CNMs are medical professionals, the overarching framework of care tends to lean toward medical, although usually at the "left" of center. CNMs own and operate a handful of freestanding birthing centers. At a midwifery birthing center, you can expect a wide range of natural methods for comfort during the birthing process, from herbal teas, showers, waterbirth tubs, herbs, and homeopathics to hypnosis techniques.

A key point of debate with freestanding birthing centers is the same point those who oppose homebirth stand on: how far will you have to go for medical help should it become necessary? Those who advocate for freestanding birthing centers are quick to note that the "distance" to help is not always something measured in time or mileage but rather has a lot more to do with the ability of the professional assisting at the birth to identify and respond to problems as they begin to unfold.

Certainly, events can turn quickly and unexpectedly, but most of the time there are enough early warning signs to raise the alert that problems could be brewing. This is why it's so important that you and your birth partner learn as much as you can about birthing and that you choose a qualified birthing professional you trust.

There's no assurance that already being in the hospital gets things done all that much faster. Hospital staff are quick to stabilize a medical situation but may be busy with someone else who's having a crisis, or there's no anesthesiologist in the hospital, or the operating rooms are all in use. For every possible problem, there are dozens of possible delays. The 20 minutes you may spend in transport are often the same 20 minutes the hospital might need to prepare for your care.

Hospital-Based Birthing Centers

Hospitals are increasing their ownership of birthing centers, driven partly by the growing demand among women for alternatives to traditional hospital births and partly by the desire to provide a broader spectrum of care and service. Some hospital birthing centers may feel quite homelike and cozy while others sneak in more clinical features such as piped-in oxygen and suction (so all the staff have to do is plug into it if it's needed, rather than bringing portable equipment into the room) and hospital-style birthing beds that are pretty hard to distinguish from genuine hospital rooms.

Some birthing centers are actually within the hospitals that own them. So instead of heading up the elevator to the fourth floor for the maternity wing, you instead turn right and go through the double glass doors that say "Birthing Center." Sometimes this arrangement is more marketing hype than measurable difference in the approach to birthing; other times you may feel that you've entered a wonderful alternate universe when those glass doors close behind you.

Not surprisingly, doctors and medically oriented nurse midwives are more comfortable assisting at births in hospital-based birthing centers. You may be more comfortable, too, if you're concerned about being close to medical services should the need for them arise. When the birthing center is in the same physical complex or right next door, staff can whisk you to a clinical setting in no time flat.

> **Trusty Midwife Tips** _____
>
> If you decide to birth at a hospital, don't go to the hospital too early! There's a prevailing belief that going to the hospital will somehow make things happen. But the opposite is more likely—whatever's happening will slow or even stop. Adrenaline starts to flow, which shuts down oxytocin—and your contractions. This sets you up for potential intervention because everyone at the hospital wants to help—and the only way they know to do this is to take action.

Ready for Anything: Hospital Birth

It's the quintessential image of impending birth: the frenetic drive or taxi ride to the hospital. Most likely, you were born in a hospital yourself. The hospital has been the primary birthing location in the United States since the end of World War II—an odd marker, to be sure, but it came about after the advent of crucial discoveries such as antibiotics and safer anesthesia that came into existence to treat battle injuries. Hospitalization and surgery for all kinds of conditions took a huge leap at the same time; it was the start of a new era in the practice of medicine.

It's not uncommon for a doctor, if that's the provider you choose, to tentatively schedule your hospital admission as you enter your second trimester of pregnancy. You probably filled out the paperwork for this during one of your first appointments, though you may not remember by now, and also paperwork authorizing the hospital to obtain any necessary approvals from your insurance company. Hospitals know well in advance that they'll fill their beds; they use this planning to determine staffing levels and other service measures. As economic factors ever-increasingly drive medical care, having your admission scheduled in advance is a lot like making an airline reservation in July for travel at Thanksgiving. Although you may be able to get the room you want if you wait, the odds are not in your favor. The hospital is the place where you're least likely to have a natural birth; you need to know this up front. Again, this is not an inherently negative aspect of birthing in the hospital; the hospital's purpose is to handle the entire spectrum of possibilities in birthing situations. But you do need to pay close attention to the hospital's presentation of its birthing approach. The more the birthing unit looks like a hospital, the more likely it functions like one, too.

When a hospital birthing unit's brochure says it supports natural birth, it means within the hospital's protocols and policies. It also often means that any vaginal birth is "natural," no matter what interventions. When you sign yourself in for care (as you will when you're admitted), you authorize the hospital and doctor to provide care deemed medically necessary. If you want a nonmedicated, nonintervention birth, your doctor may have to write specific orders to allow it. Many people—birthing women as well as their providers—find such structure comforting, and that's perfectly fine. The lines are clear; you pretty much know the decision points for interventions, and there's not much question when you cross one what the result will be.

The single-most common complaint about birthing at a hospital is the inflexibility. You must do things the hospital's way, from changing into a gown when you arrive to being in the room the hospital assigns to you to being on your back when the baby's coming. Hospital-speak focuses around the concept of "delivery"—you'll be delivered of your baby. As Chapter 2 discusses, this is about more than word play. The expectation is that others will do what needs to be done, ultimately presenting you with a baby. This does not mean that you can't have a wonderful experience giving birth in a hospital, but it does mean that ensuring a wonderful experience involves careful research into the beliefs and policies of the facility and the health-care providers working with you. No matter where or how you give birth, all birth stories are beautiful—on this, we are in full agreement!

The Business of Birthing

Nowhere in the practice of medicine (except maybe plastic surgery) is it clearer that health care is a business than when it comes to birth at hospitals. Most hospitals today are for-profit businesses (and even not-for-profits are still *in* business), and they succeed in business by making things more efficient for themselves. Time is money. A fully natural birth—no IVs, no pain meds, no fetal monitoring, no epidural, no episiotomy, no c-section—is a whole lot of nothing from the billing end of things.

Natural Woman _____

In his bestselling book *Marley and Me*, author John Grogan relates the story of his and his wife's experience with reserving the deluxe birthing suite, only to arrive to find the suite was in use. So the hospital instead put them in the "indigent care" wing where, Grogan poignantly observes, the women in labor were too poor to pay for epidurals. A recent article in *The Wall Street Journal* tallied the expense for an epidural to be nearly $3,000!

Safeguarding Your Options for Natural Birth in a Hospital

If you're considering a natural birth but want to give birth in a hospital, you really have to do your homework and prepare for all contingencies. One of the best things you could do is hire a doula (read all about doulas in Chapter 16). A doula can run interference for you and offer suggestions to help you get the birthing experience you desire. It's also important to visit the hospital's birthing unit a few times before you'll be admitted there. It's good to go on different days and times so you can see the variations in activity and staff.

Every hospital birth unit has at least one nurse who understands and supports natural birth; find out who she is and meet with her—maybe take her to coffee, if you can, so you can talk more freely. Explain what having a natural birth means to you, in terms both of the birthing experience you want and the practical sense of birthing assistance (breathing for relaxation, for example, instead of medication to make you relax). It's good for the nurse to be able to gauge your level of knowledge and understanding, too, so she knows that you know what you're talking about and have a realistic perspective of birth. Ask her what suggestions she has for you to get the birth experience you want.

Talk about fetal monitoring, IVs, and even clothing (maybe, just maybe, you'll be able to wear your own, although you're not likely to be allowed to opt for no clothing as you might at home). Talk about your anticipated birthing date, and ask the nurse about who else on the staff shares the closest philosophical position on natural birth. Also find out who you should ask for if this nurse is not there or available when you arrive. Then, when you get to the hospital for your birth, ask for this nurse by name. It's critical to get the nurses to support you, because in the hospital setting it's the nurses who run interference for the doctors.

Oh, Baby!

If you have a natural birth in a hospital, check your bill carefully—even if you have medical insurance that picks up the tab. In many hospitals, interventions such as epidurals and IVs are so commonplace that the billing form sometimes includes them automatically. Unless the doctor specifically strikes them from the billing code form, you may be charged for them.

Shifting the Energy

Want to change that frenzied hospital energy to something, well, more hospitable? Turn off the lights. Yep … just flip the switch. Hospital providers may not be used to that, so it can have the effect of stopping everyone in their tracks and may help throw off a routine mindset.

It also reminds hospital staff, "This is my birth, even though it's number 27 for you today. And today, for my birth, this is what we're going to do." Then, put on some music (you did bring your iPod or portable CD player, right?). Don't be surprised if the nurses come in and stay a while; it's calming to them, too.

> ### Trusty Midwife Tips
>
> When you do need to call in a nurse, ask specifically for the one who wants to work with nonmedicated birth. There's always at least one who's supportive of natural birth. If a nurse becomes insistent about medications or other interventions that you don't want, ask for the nurse manager—or better yet, your midwife or doctor.

A Not-So-Minor Detail: Who Pays?

Medical insurance plans typically pay for doctor and hospital expenses for a *hospital* birth, usually picking up much but not all of the costs. This is good because those costs typically add up to tens of thousands of dollars. However, you may be required to use providers that are in the insurance company's network, which means they've agreed to accept a predetermined rate of reimbursement that's less than what the provider would otherwise bill outright (like to you, if you have no medical insurance).

Coverage for a midwife, and sometimes a birthing center, can be another matter. In most states, if the insurance company will pay a doctor for a particular service, it must also pay a *nurse* midwife for the same service. Many insurance plans will also pay a certain level of coverage for a *licensed* midwife, although probably not the same percentage as for a nurse midwife. Nurse midwives, because they are within the medical model, are often included in an insurance company's provider network. Insurance companies consider midwives who are not nurses (and some who are) to be out-of-network or alternative providers, for which they pay at a lower rate.

What if your medical insurance offers only limited coverage, or does not cover at all, the provider you'd really like to choose? Before you settle for a different provider, crunch the numbers.

As insurance companies continue to shift costs, out-of-pocket expenses are climbing. Not only must you compare services and quality reports for hospitals and birthing centers you're considering, but also the costs. Most tell you what they're going to charge you during your preadmission interview, but these are estimates. A good number of women might discover that they would pay less for the services of the midwife they'd really like to use, but their insurance doesn't cover, than they'll pay for copays, deductibles, and other costs for services their insurance *does* cover. In the end, sometimes it comes down to spending a little to save a lot.

A typical hospital birth may cost $10,000 to $30,000, depending on the care you need and how long you stay. There may also be additional bills from the doctors and other providers—including the anesthesiologist if you have an epidural and any attention from specialized hospital staff. How much of this you end up on the hook for depends on your insurance coverage. By comparison, a certified midwife who attends your homebirth may charge in the neighborhood of $2,500 to $3,500 for all your prenatal visits, your birth, and your post-partum visits. You might pay the full amount out-of-pocket, but it's likely to be far less than the balance you'd owe for a hospital birth.

Deciding What Works for You

Be willing to step out of your circle of comfort during the homework phase of finding what you want. You may be surprised that what you want is not what everyone else is doing. Remember, birth is a spectrum. Sometimes the bigger challenge is discovering where you are along this spectrum and being comfortable about it.

How Likely Is a Natural Birth?	
Very likely	Homebirth with direct-entry midwife
Likely	Homebirth with nurse midwife
Somewhat likely	Hospital birth with nurse midwife
Less likely	Hospital birth with family practitioner
Unlikely	Hospital birth with an obstetrician

Give yourself permission to talk to as many people as you can—other mothers as well as providers of all kinds. From other mothers, find out how their birth experiences went and see how closely they match what you envision for yourself and your baby. The more people you talk with, the more information you'll gather about what's available and what's possible. Discuss your desires and intentions with the baby's father, if he will be part of the birth, or the birthing partner who will be present. Make sure you're on the same page when it comes to your shared vision for the birthing experience.

The Least You Need to Know

- Your choice of provider (midwife or doctor) affects your choice of location for birthing, which in turn affects your likelihood of having a natural birth.

- Homebirth offers the most intimate, private, and individual birthing experience and is just as safe as a birthing center or hospital for a routine, normal birth.

- Two of the largest medical organizations in the United States, the ACOG and the AMA, have taken official positions opposing homebirth and midwives; no other medical organizations in the world agree with these positions.

- A birthing center may offer a reasonable balance between homebirth and hospital birth, providing many of the comforts of home but with more structure and truly supporting natural birth.

- It takes considerably more effort and determination to achieve a natural birth in a hospital because the medical model of birth is inherently intervention-oriented.

Part 3

Planning for a Natural Childbirth

Birth may be the most natural experience in the world, but you have to do more than simply show up and wait for things to happen! Do you know that what you eat during your pregnancy helps shape the birth experience you'll have? Proper nutrition—and not simply eating for two—and activities that strengthen your bones and muscles as well as improve your flexibility allow your body to be in tip-top shape for the demands that birth will place on it. These chapters explore the many ways to get yourself ready for the best birth experience you and your baby can have, from a holistic perspective.

Chapter 9

What to Eat

In This Chapter

- ◆ Your body knows best when it comes to how much you should eat
- ◆ Drink like a fish (water, of course!)
- ◆ Go ahead … put a thick, lean fillet on the grill
- ◆ The hazards of restricting what and how much you eat
- ◆ Feed your labor

You already know that you need to eat well for a healthy pregnancy and a healthy baby. But you also need to eat well to have a healthy, natural birth—and not only in your final trimester, when birth preparations are on your mind, but from the first moment you know you're pregnant. (Or even before, if you're trying to have a baby.) It's never too early to lay the right foundation.

There's a lot of emphasis, and rightfully so, on eating to give your baby all the nutrients necessary for growth and development. But there's not always as much focus on meeting your own nutritional needs beyond serving the baby's needs. What you eat and drink from the start of your pregnancy plays a major role in shaping your body's ability to prepare well for birth.

Eating for You, Not Two

There's a common belief that when you're pregnant, you're eating for two. The truth of this is a technicality: keep in mind that one of that duo is only a fraction of the other's size! It's not like you and a friend are sitting down together at the table to share a nice meal. In fact, it's nothing like sharing; it's more like siphoning. Your baby takes whatever nutrients he or she needs from you right off the top of *your* nutrient stores.

When it comes to eating for your baby, you're actually replenishing what your baby has already taken from your body. Unless you're in starvation mode, your baby never goes without what she needs—but you might, if you're not keeping up. In general, your baby's drawing about 15 to 20 percent of your nutrients to meet her own needs, so that's generally how much more you need to increase what you consume yourself. This is enough to replace what the baby takes and to meet your own body's needs. But the key concept here is "general." Each woman's nutritional needs are unique.

You don't need to eat special or certain foods when you're pregnant. Like anyone else, you need to eat healthfully. The closer to "source" your foods are, the more nutritious they're likely to be. Sticking with mainly fresh fruits and vegetables, seeds and nuts, whole grains, and organic meats and poultry is one of the best ways to avoid the kinds of processed foods that are not so nutritious.

> **Trusty Midwife Tips** _____
>
> Recent studies have shown that frozen and canned vegetables and fruits have just about the same nutritional values as their fresh counterparts—just watch out for sodium (as a preservative and flavor enhancer) in vegetables and sugar ("syrup" on the label) in fruits. Eating certified organic produce and meats reduces your exposure to potentially harmful pesticides and fertilizers in produce or hormones and antibiotics in meats and poultry.

Why Calories Count ... and Why You Shouldn't Count Calories

Calories measure energy. Growing an entirely new human being takes a lot of energy. Your baby needs energy to fuel all the new construction going on in his body. His vital systems—brain and nervous system, heart and blood vessels—develop from a few cells to fully functioning networks within weeks. He nearly doubles in weight each week until about 14 weeks.

You need energy to support the many changes taking place in your own body, too. Some are changes you can see and feel, such as your enlarging breasts and swelling belly. Others are not so apparent, such as the development of new blood vessels and the increase in the amount of blood flowing through your arteries and veins. We tend to think about calories more in the context of what we take in than what we expend, but in pregnancy and birthing it's especially important to make sure you have a balance between input and output.

Don't spend a lot of effort counting calories, though. Choose a variety of foods from across the food groups. If you're truly following your body's cues, you're eating what you need to eat—and that's giving you the calories (in other words, energy) that you need, too. Counting calories when you're pregnant is no less frustrating than counting calories when you're dieting—and you don't want to get us (or you) started on that.

One problem is that when you focus on counting calories, you tend to look for ways to eat what you want (like chocolate-chip cookies) at the expense of foods that are nutritionally better for you (like apples). So go ahead, have a cookie. It won't hurt you. Later, have the apple. When you know you can have a cookie any time you want one, you find that you don't want one nearly as desperately or as often as when you think you can't have cookies.

Oh, Baby!

An unexpected and undesired consequence of attempting to limit calorie intake during pregnancy (otherwise known as dieting) is protein depletion. Even if you're eating the recommended 80 grams of protein a day, if your body needs more calories for energy than what you're consuming, eventually your body will convert the protein to energy because it's easier and faster than converting fat. As well, limiting your food intake is constipating, and you don't need anything else that creates constipation!

Focus on Nutrition, Not Weight

Pregnancy is not the time to worry about your girlish figure—or, in most cases, your weight. If you are healthy and you make nutritious eating choices, you'll gain the right amount of weight to meet your baby's needs. What's important now is that your body can supply your rapidly growing baby with the nutrients he needs to properly develop. Instead of worrying about your weight, marvel in the many changes that your body undergoes as your pregnancy progresses. There's something oddly intriguing about losing sight of your toes but gaining a look at the inside of your belly button! As much as these changes reflect the baby growing within you, they also herald your body's preparations for birthing.

If you read conventional "what to do when you're pregnant" kinds of books, you'll often find specific calorie targets for each trimester of pregnancy, framed within the context of how much weight you should gain overall (more on the weight issue later in this chapter). Some even break it out further, allocating calories according to your weight at the time you got pregnant.

With this approach, the more you weigh, the less you get to eat when you're pregnant. Hmm. Sounds rather contrary to the admonition that pregnancy is not the time to focus on weight loss, doesn't it? Your nutritional needs are pretty much the same during pregnancy no matter your weight; your body is still changing and realigning itself for nurturing as well as birthing your baby.

A more natural (and healthier) way to approach this is to simply eat when you're hungry. Eat good-quality foods, and eat them in small quantities; graze often rather than filling your plate. Such an approach puts the emphasis on getting enough of the right kinds of foods. Overeating is no better for you when you're pregnant than when you're not, but obsessing over every bite you take isn't so good for you, either.

Oh, Baby!

No matter how glamorously they're marketed, prepackaged protein drinks and "meal" smoothies aren't substitutes for the nutrients you can get from eating balanced meals and natural snacks. Bars and shakes may have a nutrient list as long as your arm, but these artificial concoctions can't provide you with the same kind of benefit you'd get from honest-to-goodness foods. And they don't taste nearly as good! The only protein drinks and snacks you should have are ones you make yourself, from real fruits, vegetables, dairy products, soy milk or tofu, and other natural protein sources.

Big Babies

Some women worry that eating too much will make a big baby. Your baby has his own agenda for growth, however. Except in certain situations (such as gestational diabetes), your baby will take from you only the nutrients he needs. It's not like he can just decide to have a second helping, because those protein molecules are sure yummy today! Big women can have big babies, certainly, but small women can have big babies, too. And usually, both can handle it just fine. Many factors contribute to your baby's size, but your weight is not usually among them.

The exception, as we alluded to, is gestational diabetes. If you have gestational diabetes, your baby has a greater likelihood of growing faster and larger than normal. This is because excess glucose is overflowing in your bloodstream, so it spills across the placenta into your baby's bloodstream. Once the glucose is in your baby's body, she has to do something with it. So she grows, and she stores more fat. Babies born to mothers who have untreated gestational diabetes can grow so large that they are unable to maneuver along the birth path. This, of course, means a c-section.

Trusty Midwife Tips

Daily physical exercise and nutritious eating habits are the most effective measures for preventing gestational diabetes, and are usually part of the treatment approach when gestational diabetes develops. Gestational diabetes may also require treatment with oral medications or insulin injections.

The Brewer Diet

In the 1970s, a San Francisco-area obstetrician named Tom Brewer (1925–2005) took a radical departure from his medical colleagues and recommended pregnant women use diet to maintain optimal health and to prevent preeclampsia. His key recommendations ran counter to conventional wisdom, such that it was:

◆ Eat 80 grams of protein, including two eggs, each day

◆ Drink at least two and preferably four quarts of water each day

◆ Salt your food to satisfy your taste

In this plan, all three components are crucial; you can't do only one or two of them. Over the years, this simple but comprehensive eating plan became the nutritional standard of natural birth. The claim that this diet can prevent preeclampsia is a source of dispute in the medical community because the causes of preeclampsia remain unknown. At the time that Dr. Brewer introduced this dietary approach, there were a number of medical interventions for preeclampsia (such as dietary restrictions and *diuretic* medications) that are

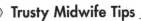

Trusty Midwife Tips

Many of the books written by Dr. Tom Brewer and Gail Sforza Brewer are now out of print. However, copies are still available through used book sellers, and the sharing network—libraries and borrowing from people who have copies of the book—is alive and well.

today no longer used because, as Dr. Brewer believed, they did not prevent preeclampsia and often caused other problems. However, there is no dispute that eating nutritiously is one of the best things you can do to maintain optimal health for yourself and your baby.

> **Birthing Book** _____
>
> A **diuretic** is a substance that causes the body to increase its excretion of fluid. In other words, it makes you pee more. A diuretic may be in the form of a medication (such as hydrochlorothiazide or furosemide) or a naturally occurring substance (such as dandelion, nettle, or watermelon). Caffeine and sugar also have diuretic effects.

Beef (or Bean) Up the Protein

Might a steak a day keep the doctor away? Odds are good! During your pregnancy, your body needs protein—lots of it. Your blood volume is going to increase to half again what it is when you're not pregnant to carry all those new red blood cells, which in turn carry iron and oxygen. That's pretty substantial—and about 80 percent of that increase is in albumin, the protein-based fluid that transports blood cells through your arteries and veins. Albumin gives your blood its volume; blood volume allows your body to maintain pressure within your blood vessels. This is essential for life. You also need protein to repair cells and allow new cells to grow.

Your body can get the protein it needs to make more albumin (a task your liver handles) only from dietary sources—the foods you eat. You need about 60 to 80 grams of protein every day when you're pregnant. This is half again to twice as much protein as would otherwise be healthy; your nonpregnant body needs only 30 to 40 grams of protein daily. If you already eat a lot of meat or legumes (such as lentils and soy-based foods) every day, you may not have to make much of a change in your eating habits.

Most women, especially those following a vegetarian or vegan lifestyle, don't eat enough protein even when they're not pregnant. When your body needs protein, it craves meat. Don't be surprised if you find yourself lunging across the table to take someone else's chicken breast! Sometimes your baby will demand a change in diet, or your own tastes will change. The urge for meat usually goes away after the baby is born, though.

Protein has the added advantage of making you feel full faster and longer. Although most foods, even fruits and vegetables, contain some protein, the best sources are meats, legumes such as lentils, and soy products such as tofu. Some foods that are high in protein are also high in fat, so it's important to read labels and assess the nutritional content. Some of the healthier choices may surprise you, such as steak (a lean cut, of course). Remember, a healthy portion size fits in the palm of your hand.

If you are vegetarian or vegan, you may need to increase your protein consumption slowly to allow your digestive system to adjust. Plant-based foods that are high in protein are often also high in fiber, which can make you quite gassy.

Are you worried about soy as a source of protein? There are some who question whether soy, as a phytoestrogen, affects the development of the baby's sex organs. Research studies involving rats don't hold up very well against centuries of soy-based diets in countries such as Japan and China. Most health experts believe dietary soy poses no health risks to the developing baby and offers many health benefits for the mother, especially if it's organic.

Adequate protein is especially important for helping your body maintain a healthy blood pressure and to prevent preeclampsia, a potentially dangerous rise in blood pressure toward the end of the third trimester. (Chapter 3 discusses preeclampsia.)

Here are some foods that are high in protein (and remember: organic is best):

- turkey (the most protein per serving)
- beef (choose lean cuts)
- pork (choose lean cuts)
- chicken (choose breast meat)
- eggs (especially whites)
- fish
- soybeans (edamame)

- soybean products such as tofu
- lentils
- beans (navy, pinto, white, kidney)
- cheese
- yogurt
- milk
- raw nuts and seeds

Oh, Baby!

Should you worry about mercury and other heavy metal contamination in fish? Health experts do recommend that you limit to six ounces or less per week, or even avoid eating altogether, certain kinds of fish—albacore tuna, mackerel, and swordfish—during pregnancy because these fish tend to live in environments where heavy metal pollution is more concentrated, so they accumulate particularly high levels in their tissues. Heavy metals such as mercury and lead can have damaging effects on your baby's developing brain and nervous system.

Keep It Real

The foods that give you the most nutrients are those that you can identify as having a place in the natural world—fruits, vegetables, whole grains, nuts, meats, poultry, and fish. Real chickens don't have nuggets; fish aren't square; carrots have dimples and root hairs; and broccoli looks like bonsai. If you start to get confused, think about what you'd like to see your baby eating. That's what you should have.

Sometimes it's difficult to eat as much as you should when you're pregnant. Early in pregnancy, you may have morning sickness that sends you dashing for the bathroom at the mere sight, smell, or even thought of certain foods. Late in pregnancy, your baby's taking up a lot of room in your belly and may be pressing against your stomach. You may feel full all the time, even when you don't eat. Smaller meals more often, and even snacks every few hours, may help you work around this situation.

Trusty Midwife Tips

About half of pregnant women experience morning sickness, which researchers believe results from the rapid changes in hormones during the first trimester of pregnancy. There are many natural remedies to help calm your queasies; among them are ginger root (found in real ginger ale—you have to read the label) and the smell of peppermint. Acupressure is also very effective for many women (see Chapter 11).

Drink Up!

Your body is working to bring on board enough fluid that your ligaments, tendons, muscles, and other tissues are able to stretch and loosen as they need to for your baby to pass down the birth path. You may feel thirstier than usual or find that you want more to drink even if you don't actually feel thirsty. This is your body telling you to pump up the liquids.

During your pregnancy, you should drink two to four quarts of water every day. And water means water, not juice, soda, tea, or coffee. Sugar in drinks such as sodas and juices takes three times as much water to process. So for every 12-ounce can of soda you consume, you need to drink three 12-ounce glasses of water to get the right amount of fluid into your body. As well, tea and coffee (and some sodas) contain caffeine, which has a diuretic action—actually drawing more fluid from your body than you're putting in. You're much better off to just drink water!

When you're not adequately hydrated, your body's balance of essential salts (electrolytes) gets distorted. Your body falls into rescue mode, attempting to entice you to drink more. You may find that you crave salt and salty foods; eating salty foods causes you to feel thirsty and to feel that you need to drink. Staying adequately hydrated also boosts your energy level, helping you feel more alert and able to concentrate. Hydration becomes critical during labor. A body that's dehydrated, even a little bit, makes labor hurt more and take longer. No one wants to be in that category! So drink up.

Your blood volume, as we said earlier, increases by about half during your pregnancy to improve your blood's ability to carry oxygen and nutrients for your baby. Hydration is important in this process. However, many beverages and some foods contain substances that act as *diuretics*—they draw fluid out of your body. This can result in dehydration, even though you're drinking the recommended amounts of liquids. Here are some common substances that have diuretic action:

- caffeine
- alcohol
- sugar
- herbal/botanical ingredients: dandelion, alfalfa, bilberry, nettle
- celery

- parsley
- asparagus
- watermelon
- excessive quantities of water-soluble vitamins (B vitamins, vitamin C)

Eating During Labor

If birthing is the most intense physical activity you'll ever do, you need plenty of nourishment—food and water—to stay strong and focused. Yet the conventional practice in hospitals and many birthing centers is to withhold food and drink! The rationale, of course, is that you may need a c-section, in which case having a full gut is dangerous because you might *aspirate* if you need *intubation* for the administration of general anesthesia. So instead, you can have an IV that trickles fluid (mostly water) into your veins. Not quite the same. Your body really wants and needs to get its water by having you drink it, which is its normal path of hydration—not through an IV.

For a successful natural birth, you need to eat and drink as you feel like doing. A bowl of soup or a cup of hot tea can refresh both your body and your spirits, as can having your midwife feed you a slice of pizza while you're standing in the shower at 9 centimeters along in your labor. Eating and drinking are acts of comfort as much as of nourishment. You're more likely to feel queasy when you don't eat, even if there is an IV in your arm. If you drink and eat at will, you're the one in charge of getting the proper energy and fluid into your body—which is as it should be.

> **Trusty Midwife Tips**
>
> If you're using a birthing tub during labor, it's especially important to take regular drinks of water or juice to keep yourself well hydrated. Being in the warm water draws fluid from your body, although you're not usually aware of it. If you feel thirsty, you're not drinking enough. Put a couple small tables next to the birthing tub so you can always have something to drink within easy reach, without the need to ask someone to get a drink for you. Water bottles for sporting activities are often good for this purpose because they're contoured or have no-slip features, making them easier to hold on to when your hands are wet.

The Least You Need to Know

- Your body needs additional protein and water when you're pregnant so its tissues can soften and loosen in preparation for birthing.

- Eat often, eat small portions, and eat real food.

- Getting enough protein, water, and salt is crucial for maintaining your body's fluid balance and blood pressure and to possibly prevent preeclampsia.

- Eating and drinking are acts of self-comfort as much as routes of nourishment.

- Staying well-hydrated during labor helps you stay comfortable and keeps your labor progressing.

Chapter 10

Yoga, Stretching, and Massage

In This Chapter

◆ Relaxin: another hormone getting your body ready

◆ Yoga: uniting mind, body, and spirit

◆ Stretching for flexibility

◆ The comfort of touch: massage

Your body has to make some major adjustments and accommodations for birthing. It's pretty amazing, really, that your body has the ability to flex, stretch, and loosen in ways that open a birth path for your baby. You can work with this ability to further prepare for birthing by using a blend of ancient and modern methods to gently stretch and strengthen the tissues and muscles that participate in the birthing process.

Increasing your flexibility extends your breathing capacity, too. Methods such as yoga emphasize the breath beyond simply breathing in and breathing out and will be very helpful to you during labor and birth, even if you take traditional birth education classes that teach breathing techniques for labor.

Relaxin' with Relaxin

Among the many changes taking place in your body as your pregnancy advances are the loosening and softening of connective tissues throughout your body. The substance most responsible for these changes is a hormone called, appropriately, *relaxin*. So, if you find yourself dropping the milk just handed to you and you feel more klutzy than usual, it's because relaxin is everywhere. Although these changes affect all your joints, it's your pelvis that's most profoundly altered. During birth, this looseness lets your pelvic joints separate and widen to allow your baby's passage from your uterus and along the birth path.

> **Birthing Book**
>
> Relaxin is a hormone your placenta produces during pregnancy that causes connective tissue in your body to soften and loosen, allowing broader flexibility of your joints. Relaxin is normally present in your body in small amounts and greatly increases during pregnancy.

Remember in Chapter 4, we talked about how your cervix actually moves around during your menstrual cycle? The corpus luteum, a yellowish structure that remains in the ovarian follicle after the release of an egg (ovulation), produces a burst of relaxin as the egg is traveling through your fallopian tube. The burst lasts just about as long as the period of time that you're fertile to give your ordinarily firm cervix the ability to soften, relax, and shift slightly forward. This is like throwing open the door and turning on the light to welcome any sperm that may come calling. And for added good measure, semen contains relaxin, too.

In a menstrual cycle when there is no conception, the corpus luteum shrinks away, relaxin drops off, and your cervix returns to its normal position. Your breasts do continue to make small amounts of relaxin that remain in your system, helping keep your joints and connective tissues (ligaments, tendons, and fascia) supple. When you become pregnant, however, first your corpus luteum and then your placenta step in to take over relaxin production, churning out especially copious amounts of it in your first trimester (another of relaxin's functions is to spur the growth of new blood vessels, called angiogenesis, such as those that attach the placenta to your uterus) and again as labor begins (preparing your body for the baby's birth). The corpus luteum hangs out during the first trimester and does this work until the placenta gets established toward the end of the first trimester, then the placenta picks up the task. Relaxin levels return to normal shortly after the baby is born.

> **Trusty Midwife Tips**
>
> The relaxin that softens your connective tissues affects the walls of your veins, too. This makes it easier to develop varicose veins, including the dreaded hemorrhoids (varicose veins in the rectum). Toe stretches, along with walking and swimming, help keep muscles firm and supportive around the veins in your legs. Do them in the shower—raise yourself onto your toes, then lower yourself back down. The warm water is soothing, and you can put your hands on the shower wall for support.

Yoga: As One

Yoga dates back to ancient India and is a holistic practice that blends physical movement with mental focus. The word yoga comes from Sanskrit and means "yoke"—to join together in unity and harmony. The usual connotation in the practice of yoga is the integration of body, mind, and spirit. In pregnancy, there's the added dimension of the partnership between you and your baby.

In modern usage, a yoke is a device that holds two animals, usually oxen or cattle, together such that they must learn to move in perfect unison to move at all. Setting aside the intimation of subservience, this is an interesting context because the idea in the practice of yoga is to so completely unify your mental focus (thoughts) and movement (body) that they always happen together through postures (also called poses) that require such unison and concentration. In ancient India, "yuj," the origin of the word yoga, meant "to control." Discipline, which blends control and focus, is at the core of yoga's philosophy. This is exactly what needs to happen during birth.

Despite such solemn origins, the best thing about yoga is that it makes you feel great! Yoga is a wonderful way to relax, re-center yourself, and tune in to your body while tuning out distracting thoughts, worries, and fears. If you're already a yogini, keep doing what you're doing (with the appropriate modifications when necessary, of course).

If you're new to yoga, start with a class. Most metropolitan areas have an abundance of yoga offerings, including special classes for pregnant women; many small communities and even rural areas often have at least someone who practices yoga and does group sessions once or twice a week. If formal classes are not available at all for you, there's a wealth of information on the web. DVDs that lead yoga for pregnant women are another option. Look for yoga teachers who have good credentials and whose teaching approach and yoga method are comfortable for you, and who either are teaching classes specifically for pregnant women or have experience teaching yoga for pregnant women.

The Breath

The breath—not just breathing but also the breath itself—is critically important in yoga. The breath is the life energy in many Eastern practices, a vital and dynamic force rather than something to be held, and yoga is no exception. The Sanskrit word for the breath in this context is *prana*.

> **Birthing Book**
>
> **Prana** is the Sanskrit word for breath, which in ancient cultures was an entity in its own right, separate from organs such as the lungs. Prana also connotes life force or life energy.

Focusing your awareness on the breath as you breathe causes you to stay in the moment of now—not the moment that just was and not the moment that's coming next. Your breath gets your full and conscious attention. It's hard to be anxious, scared, or worried when your focus is on your breath.

Nearly instantly you can feel yourself relax and calm down. When you practice yoga breathing on a regular and frequent basis, the calming becomes preventive—you stay centered in yourself, and all the outside static passes you by.

Yoga views breathing as having three levels: high or clavicle (collarbone) breathing, middle or rib-cage breathing, and low or belly breathing. High breathing uses mainly the top part of your lungs and feels shallow. Middle breathing expands your rib cage to pull air deeper into your lungs. And low breathing draws air low into your body, fully engaging your diaphragm and abdominal muscles.

By your third trimester and into labor, your natural breathing pattern is high breathing because your baby's pressing against your diaphragm—and your big belly causes you to lean forward when you sit, stand, and walk. If you often feel breathless, little wonder! But you have more red blood cells in your blood now, too, and they're all lined up in there like railroad cars—eager to pick up more oxygen molecules and deliver them all through your body and to your baby. So focusing on your breath also helps you get more oxygen into your blood.

Exercises for the breath are called pranayama. The following sections lead you through three pranayama that are easy to learn and do: basic (easy) breathing, complete (three-part) breathing, and alternate nostril breathing. Once you master them, you can do them anywhere. It's good to practice them often so they become second nature for you. Then they'll come naturally when you need them, such as when you're birthing.

Basic (Easy) Breathing

1. Sit comfortably and with enough support that you can hold your spine tall—not stretching but not slouching, either. All parts of your body should be open and relaxed—feet on the floor, arms at your sides, palms facing upward. If you need to put a pillow under your sit bones to feel comfortable sitting on the floor in a true upright posture, go ahead and do that; use the pillow as a wedge (don't just sit on it!). As your pregnancy advances, it may be harder to sit on the floor; don't worry about it. Find a straight-backed chair and use that. The point is to sit in a manner that elongates your spine without pulling it out of alignment.

2. Become aware of your breath moving through your nostrils and in and out of your body. Just feel it without trying to control it, but giving it your full attention.

3. Fully experience your breath—how it feels, how it sounds, how it smells. Feel your breath fill your lungs, linger, and then leave your lungs. Experience how your breath feels as it leaves your body.

Keep your focus entirely on your breath. If your thoughts start to wander, bring them back to your breath. Do Basic Breathing for six to ten cycles of breathing (breathe in, breathe out equals one cycle). Make sure to breathe only through your nostrils, not your mouth. Basic Breathing is a good way to restore your sense of well-being and reconnect with your body during labor. You can do it as frequently as you like and in any position that makes you comfortable.

Complete (Three-Part) Breathing

1. Sit comfortably and with enough support that you can hold your spine tall— not stretching but not slouching, either. All parts of your body should be open and relaxed—feet on the floor, arms at your sides, and palms facing upward. If you can sit on the floor, that's great. If your pregnancy is far enough along that you're not comfortable on the floor, use a straight-backed chair.

2. Take two or three deep breaths and exhale completely after each, as cleansing breaths. Breathe in and out only through your nostrils.

3. Begin to breathe in, focusing on the breath. Feel the breath fill your body from the bottom (your belly) up, like pouring water into a glass. Keep your breathing steady.

4. When the breath fills you to your collarbones, begin to breathe out. Feel the breath leave your body from the top down, like pouring water out of a glass. Keep your breathing steady and empty your lungs completely.

5. Repeat for three to five cycles, keeping your full focus on the breath as it moves in and out of your body.

Complete Breathing expands your chest and upper body to let more air into your lungs. This increases the amount of oxygen entering your blood circulation. Keep your breathing steady and paced; if you begin to feel lightheaded, you're breathing too fast (hyperventilating) and not focusing on the breath. If this happens, pause to refocus your thoughts on your breath, then return to finish the cycles. Complete Breathing is especially balancing and invigorating in labor and is great to do when you're in a birthing tub and the water takes much of the pressure away from your body.

Complete Breathing also helps keep your fingers and hands from falling asleep toward the end of your pregnancy. Some women really feel this when lying down. When everything's all scrunched up in your torso, as it gets toward the end of pregnancy, the nerves coming from your spine get pinched. Straightening the alignment of your vertebrae, as Complete Breathing helps you to do, releases the pinching and stops the tingling.

Alternate Nostril Breathing

1. Sit comfortably and with enough support that you can hold your spine tall—not stretching but not slouching, either. All parts of your body should be open and relaxed—feet on the floor, arms at your sides, and palms facing upward. If you can sit on the floor, that's great. If your pregnancy is far enough along that you're not comfortable on the floor, use a straight-backed chair.

2. Take two or three deep breaths and exhale completely after each as cleansing breaths. Breathe in and out only through your nostrils.

3. Press your right nostril closed with your right index finger. Breathe in and out through your left nostril, focusing on the experience of the breath moving in and out of your body. Keep your breathing steady and measured (not fast, not slow) and at the same pace breathing in and breathing out. Repeat for three to five cycles of breathing.

4. Release your right nostril and press your left nostril closed with your left index finger. Breathe in and out through your right nostril, again focusing on the experience of the breath moving in and out of your body. Keep your breathing steady and measured. Repeat for the same number of cycles you did with your right nostril.

5. Release your left nostril. Take two or three steady, measured breaths through both nostrils to return to normal breathing.

The ancient yogis believed Alternate Nostril Breathing restored balance in the flow of the breath through the body and especially to the brain. They observed that during natural breathing, the nostrils alternate dominance with one taking the lead and then the other. However, the nostrils do not naturally balance themselves, so one may be dominant longer than the other.

The yogis also correlated nostril dominance with brain function, perceiving the left nostril to bring in breath that supports intuition and creativity and the right nostril to bring in breath that supports reason and logic. Not surprisingly, scientific research studies have recently confirmed these observations. Breathing longer on one side allows those traits to dominate—so if your right nostril is taking control, you may feel agitated and nervous because your logical brain is trying to overmanage things.

When you use Alternate Nostril Breathing to restore balance, your intuitive brain can again step into the picture and help restore your faith in your ability to birth. Some yoga practitioners believe air flowing into the left nostril creates calm and peace and air flowing into the right nostril is invigorating and motivates immediate action, much as adrenaline does. Try it!

Poses

A yoga pose, or posture, is called an asana. Yoga poses integrate the body and the breath through concentration. Many yoga poses move from one pose to another. Your yoga class (or session, if you're doing it alone) should start with some gentle movements and breathing exercises to get your body warmed up and ready. Always move into yoga poses slowly and smoothly, and stop if something feels not quite right. While your relaxed ligaments, tendons, and joints make it easier for you to be flexible, you're also more vulnerable to doing too much and causing injury.

Oh, Baby!

Your center of balance is ever shifting as your pregnancy advances. Yoga poses that are easy in your second trimester may become impossible in your third trimester. Learn a variety of poses so you always have some from which to choose.

Use modified poses when traditional poses are too challenging or strenuous. A good yoga instructor knows how to help people use modified poses that accommodate whatever physical constraints they have, and a yoga instructor who teaches prenatal yoga knows specifically what works best when you're pregnant. From the second trimester on, avoid yoga poses in which you're flat on your back. Your heavy belly can compress blood vessels and nerves, leading to unpleasant sensations and possible problems.

Always remember: if it doesn't feel right, don't do it. Your intuition is never wrong. You want to make things easier for your body, not stress it. This is not the time to push yourself in that way. Yoga isn't about pain or pushing beyond what the body is able (and willing) to do. If it hurts, you've gone too far. Listening to your body is part of the concentration that yoga provides; the more you listen, the more you hear. During birth, you'll appreciate this kind of concentration, and your yoga practice will help make it more natural to you.

Here are some good yoga poses for pregnancy and labor:

- **Cat Pose (Marjariasana):** A kneeling pose that arches your full spine. Because your belly hangs down, Cat Pose helps relieve low back discomfort.

- **Cobbler's Pose (Boddha Konasana):** Also called Bound Angle Pose, this seated pose opens the hips and pelvis and stretches the upper legs. Cobbler's Pose is especially effective in the last trimester of pregnancy, and can improve comfort with contractions in early labor.

- **Cow Pose (Bitilasana):** A kneeling pose that flexes your full spine. Like Cat Pose, Cow Pose is great for back discomfort. Cow Pose and Cat Pose are often combined.

- **Downward-Facing Dog Pose (Adho Mukha Svanasana):** A forward-bending pose best done with your partner's help, Downward-Facing Dog stretches the lower back, glutes, hamstrings, calves, Achilles, and plantar surfaces of the feet. It can become difficult to get into and out of this pose in late pregnancy.

- **Firelog Pose (Agnistambhasana):** The seated Firelog Pose opens and stretches the hips, and is more challenging than some of the other poses. Firelog Pose is also helpful for sciatica and insomnia.

◆ **Lion Pose (Simhasana):** Another seated pose, Lion Pose is especially effective for relieving tension in the neck and jaw.

◆ **Pigeon Pose (Eka Pada Rajakapotasana):** Pigeon Pose stretches the glutes and groin muscles, and flexes the hips. It begins on all fours.

◆ **Side Plank Pose (Vasisthasana):** A balance pose, the Side Plank Pose strengthens the arms and the body's core. In pregnancy it's often necessary to modify the Side Plank Pose by extending a foot for counterbalance.

◆ **Staff Pose (Dandasana):** The seated Staff Pose stretches the legs, especially the quads, and opens the spine.

◆ **Tiger Pose (Vyaghrasana):** Tiger Pose is a stretching pose done on all fours. It opens the spine, pelvis, and neck and shoulders.

◆ **Triangle Pose (Utthita Trikonasana):** Triangle Pose is a standing pose that stretches the hamstrings and opens the chest and shoulders. As your belly gets bigger, you may need to modify the stretch.

◆ **Warrior Poses (Virabhadrasana I and II):** The Warrior Poses are standing poses that open the chest and spine, stretch the legs and arms, and strengthen the body core.

Trusty Midwife Tips

New to yoga, or need to know how to adapt these and other yoga poses for your changing body and balance? Google the pose on the web to locate pictures and video clips for illustration and guidance. Some popular sites include www.healthandyoga.com, aboutyoga.com, and www.yoga.com. You can also check out *The Complete Idiot's Guide to Yoga Illustrated, Fourth Edition* by Joan Budilovsky, Ph.D., and Eve Adamson.

Yoga in Labor and Birthing

Yoga breathing techniques are especially helpful during labor because they shift your focus from your body to your breath. The calming effect on your thoughts is nearly instant, and your body is again free to do what it knows how to do. When you can go with the flow of your breath, you also can go with the flow of your body. You can use yoga breathing techniques in any position that makes you comfortable in labor and birthing. Your baby also gets the message that all is well and can continue to help with the labor and birth.

Many women find yoga poses can relieve pressure and discomfort during labor. Poses that are on all fours with the belly down, such as Cat Pose and Cow Pose, are especially helpful with any pressure you feel in your lower back. Modified Triangle Pose and the Warrior Poses can help you flex and stretch your spine and back. And the Lion Pose may release you to roar like a lioness as well as open your pelvis.

Stretches: Range of Motion

Conventional stretching and range of motion movements are also very helpful during pregnancy, labor, and birthing, although they have more of a medical orientation to them or an athletic orientation, if you've been active in sports like running and cycling. As with yoga, it's important to coordinate breathing with physical movements.

People sometimes hold their breath when stretching; this is counterproductive. Steady breathing helps keep your movements steady and also gets much-needed oxygen into your blood. This is important because you're asking your muscles to work, and they need oxygen both to fuel their efforts and to help carry away the metabolic byproducts of their activity.

Stretching Routine

A typical stretching routine may start from the toes and work up your body to your head. You can begin seated or standing. If you stand, have a chair, countertop, or wall nearby that you can use for balance and support. Keep all your movements gentle, measured, and smooth.

1. Start by slightly raising one leg and wiggling your toes.

2. Let the movement spread up your leg, flexing and rotating your ankle and then your knee.

> **Trusty Midwife Tips**
>
> Make sure your muscles are warm when you begin stretching. Warm muscles have plenty of blood bringing them vital oxygen, which makes them receptive to stretching and activity. It helps to be in a warm environment, too.

3. Extend your hip to the front, back, and side.

4. Move your pelvis forward, back, and side to side.

5. Wiggle the fingers on the same side.

6. Flex and rotate your wrist and then your elbow. Extend your arm out, back, and up to flex and stretch your shoulder.

7. Finally, rotate your neck slowly and as fully as is comfortable.

8. Move back down the same side of your body, reversing the order until you're back at your toes.

9. Do the other side.

You can do this stretching routine as often as you like throughout the day, and it's also helpful during labor. Stretching can also be passive, with your partner or midwife moving your muscles and joints through the stretching motions while you're sitting or lying down.

Let the Water Carry You Away

Gentle swim strokes are great for stretching and toning your muscles and connective tissues. Being in the water removes three fourths of gravity's pull, letting you move with ease in ways that are difficult—if not impossible—on land. You can even be belly-down—when was the last time you could do that? In the water, you can be comfortable in just about any position.

Swim strokes work the range of motion for nearly every joint in your body, without stress or strain. Do them slowly, such that you glide rather than splash through the water. Focus on the flow of your breath as it fills your lungs and spreads through your fluid body. Envision tiny bubbles of air emerging from the tips of your toes as you kick through the water, giving your entire being buoyancy and lightness.

Feel the strong, smooth movements of your muscles as you complete each stroke cycle. Give yourself over to the primal solitude of being in the water. When your face is in the water, envision your baby floating in the safe pool of amniotic fluid within your womb. Let the water bond you through this shared experience of being submerged. Here are some common swim strokes and the unique ways each might benefit you.

- The breaststroke opens your chest, abdomen, shoulder girdle, and pelvic girdle. The wide, pulling arm stroke puts your shoulders through nearly a complete range of motion cycle. The standard whip-kick (or the old-school frog-kick) does the same for your hips and also your knees and ankles. The top of each stroke fully extends your torso, widening your rib cage. Concentrate on a smooth, flowing stroke without jerky movements—even if you need to soften your kick to do so.

- Freestyle (or crawl) also stretches your shoulder girdle and torso but without so much pelvic action. Instead, your body can gently twist from side to side, flexing your spine. Kick from the hip to protect your knees, and pull your toes forward with each kick-stroke to flex your ankles (although this isn't quite correct technique).

◆ Sidestroke, with its alternating arm stroke and gentle scissors kick, is relaxing and low stress. Your belly makes this stroke easier, balancing the movements of your arms and legs. Switch sides to give both sides of your body equal effort.

◆ If lying on your back is a challenge most of the time, the backstroke takes the pressure off. Your large belly may make it difficult for you to get enough arch in your back to support this stroke (and it makes other people smile to see it sticking above the water), but the back rotation of the arm stroke can really open up your shoulders and your chest.

Trusty Midwife Tips _____

Make sure to drink plenty of water when you're swimming. Being in the water doesn't keep you from becoming dehydrated, and because you're in the water you may not feel thirsty. It's a good idea to have a water bottle poolside so you can take a few swigs every 15 minutes or so. After your swim, drink a full 12 ounces of water.

Swimming is particularly valuable for opening and relaxing your upper body. Although of course you're not going to break out into a gracious breaststroke during labor, swimming once or twice a week during your last trimester really limbers your shoulders and torso. During labor and birthing, this will help you greatly with breathing and getting good amounts of oxygen to your baby (as well as into your body for your own use). Exhaling underwater automatically increases your lung capacity. Hydrostatic pressure is greater that atmospheric pressure, so it's actually harder work to blow bubbles underwater than to blow bubbles in the air.

Stretching During Labor and Birthing

Stretching helps to relieve sore or stiff muscles during labor. Sometimes you spend too much time in one position during the course of your day, causing discomfort. You can do selected segments of stretching, depending on how you feel and the position you're in.

You may be most comfortable on all fours but feel tension in your shoulders and neck, so do the stretching movements for your upper body to relax and relieve this physical stress. Or get something to support your upper body to relieve the tension in that part of your body. Stretching during labor also helps you keep your torso and upper body open so you can breathe more deeply, bringing more oxygen into your blood circulation. Your partner can help by supporting your arm or leg as you do the stretches, even adding some gentle massage if that helps you feel better.

Doing stretches while you're in the birthing tub isn't quite the same as swimming, but the water does reduce the resistance that gravity imposes on movement. Stretch, rock your hips, and move your arms back and forth on the surface of the water. Keep the movements steady and smooth as if you were in a pool.

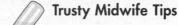

Trusty Midwife Tips

Feeling the strain of carrying your bulging belly as your pregnancy advances? Have your partner (or anyone you wish) stand behind you, reach around with both hands, and gently "hold" your belly up for a few minutes. What a relief!

Massage: Hands On

Massage is great during pregnancy and also during labor because it not only relaxes and soothes muscles, it also causes your body to release those feel-good endorphins. You can have someone else massage you, such as a massage therapist, or learn massage techniques you can do yourself. A massage from a massage therapist will specifically target muscle groups to loosen any tightness and to increase circulation to them.

Oh, Baby!

Massage releases toxins stored in your muscles, which can be a load on your liver as it works to break them down. It's essential to drink all the water the massage therapist tells you that you need to drink to help safely flush these substances from your body.

Ah, That Feels Good!

Touch, especially from someone you love and trust, feels good. It conveys calm and confidence—the sense that everything is fine. Even when you know this, it's good to feel it through someone else's hands. Having someone else (especially your partner) massage your lower back, your shoulders, your arms, your legs, and even your belly can be very soothing and relaxing.

Don't be shy about saying what you like and don't like when someone else is massaging you. You may find that what feels good and what makes you want to leap right off the massage table is likely to change. Pregnancy hormones have many affects on your senses, especially touch (your skin) and smell (massage oil fragrances). You do want to use an oil with a massage, but you can use something such as olive oil or grapeseed oil. The oil softens and warms the skin and lubricates the touch.

Many massage therapists have been taught that there are certain uterine points along the lower legs which, if stimulated by massage, will cause labor to begin or intensify. The body certainly has its mysteries, but think about it. If truly this were possible and a massage therapist or anyone else could touch these points and get that baby to shoot out, there'd never be an issue about inducing labor! Not only that … massage therapists would be the most highly paid people on the planet. Although this has long been disproven, it remains embedded in common wisdom—and a good number of massage therapists won't touch the legs of a pregnant woman.

Self-Massage

You can massage parts of your body yourself, although sometimes your focus is elsewhere or you can't quite reach the parts that ache (such as your back or your lower legs). The advantage is that you know exactly where you are tight or the muscles are sore, and you can target them with motions that bring you instant relief. Self-massage is particularly effective when you first become aware that an area is becoming stiff, so you can keep it from becoming painful.

Perineal Massage

Massaging the perineal area to increase its ability to stretch is controversial. Perineal massage became popular as an approach to reducing the need for episiotomy. Allowing the birth to take its time and waterbirth are unquestionably the best ways to let the perineal tissues naturally open without tearing. Setting that aside, however, perineal massage *before* birthing may help soften the perineal tissues. Perineal massage *during* birthing—especially during crowning, as had become popular a few years ago—may be more likely to result in perineal tears. Don't mess with anything as the baby emerges!

The perineum is very sensitive anyway, and during birthing it's on a clear mission of its own. Touching it in any way is very likely to alter the hormone surges that are pushing the baby along the birth path—even to the extent of halting the contraction. Perineal tissue is normally pink. If it turns white, it's stretching too fast and is at risk for tearing.

This is when the midwife or partner should tell the woman, "Stop and just let your body do it all with no efforts to help." This will let the baby's head move back just a bit to take the pressure off the perineal tissue. This backing and forthing of the baby's head during crowning is what allows the tissue to open and accommodate the size without tearing.

Many childbirth education programs do recommend prenatal perineal massage, done toward the end of the third trimester. This is usually something your partner does, although some women can do it for themselves. It's important to learn the correct method so you get the intended stretching effect. Otherwise, it's just a lot of rubbing (and not a lot of fun).

There is a device, not available in the United States but used in many other countries, that is inserted into the vagina and gradually expanded to simulate the size of a baby's head. The idea is to get your tissues and your mind familiar with how this feels. The issue, though, is that when this happens for real, you have all kinds of hormones to soften your tissues and otherwise prepare your body for this event. Chapters 18 and 19 talk much more about crowning, perineal stretching, and the birth process.

Massage During Labor and Birthing

Many women find massage to be enormously comforting and relaxing during labor and birthing; other women prefer to be totally focused within themselves and don't want to be touched at all. Some women want to be touched; then they don't. Whatever works for you is what's right, so don't be concerned that you should let someone massage your back when really all you want is to get in the birthing tub and breathe.

Do tell your partner, midwife, or doula if you'd like them to massage your back, shoulders, or feet. This is all about you, after all, and they won't know what feels best to you unless you tell them. Sometimes you may want to combine stretching and massage, which is fine.

The Least You Need to Know

- The hormone relaxin helps prepare your body for birth by relaxing and softening your muscles and ligaments.

- Yoga's breathing exercises and poses improve your ability to focus and your flexibility.

- Massage is a great way to involve your partner in helping you stay comfortable.

- Swimming helps you stretch your muscles, improve the range of motion of your joints, and expand the ability of your lungs to take in air.

Chapter 11

Preparing for a Mindful Birth

In This Chapter

- Shining the light of mindfulness on your fears and worries
- Getting back to, and staying in, the moment
- Keeping a lid on cortisol
- Using mindfulness and breathing exercises for comfort during labor
- Other methods to reach the subconscious: energy work

It's well documented that mindfulness helps you stay relaxed and calm within your body. Your breathing is regular and efficient. Mindfulness techniques can help you be comfortable during labor. They also can help you deal with your worries, fears, and other emotional issues throughout your pregnancy, too, so when the time for birthing arrives, you're confident and looking forward to both the experience of birthing and to meeting your baby.

There's nothing elaborate or mystical about mindfulness—anyone can do it, anywhere, and at any time. All you have to do is allow your thoughts, feelings, and emotions to exist without judgment or control. Sounds easy enough, doesn't it?

Thought Bubbles: An Exercise in Mindfulness

What worries or scares you the most about the birthing experience that lies ahead? Maybe there are lots of things; just allow one to come forward for right now, and you can use mindfulness to work your way through the others later.

Mindfulness is especially beneficial for helping you to examine and get to the bottom of things that worry, trouble, or scare you. Sometimes the feelings these things evoke are intense and unpleasant, and we do just about anything we can to avoid them and bury them deep in the subconscious part of the brain. Of course, this doesn't make these fears go away, and they continue to affect us.

Here's a short mindfulness exercise. Start by making yourself comfortable. Sit or lie down in an open, unrestricted position, with your arms and legs uncrossed. Take a few slow, deep breaths in and out to let your body relax. Let the fear rise to the surface of your mind like a thought bubble. As that bubble's bobbing around, take a closer look at it. Shine a light on it. You can see it from all sides, even underneath and behind, because it's a bubble. Form no judgment about it, just explore it. Now, does it still scare you so much? How do you feel?

Much better, isn't it? You've noticed a thought, and instead of trying to banish it because it scares you or you don't think you should be thinking it, you've given that elusive thought your focused attention. You've authenticated its existence—because it *does* exist, even if you choose (or try) to ignore it. You've allowed the thought to simply be, without trying to do anything with it, to it, or about it. This, in a nutshell, is mindfulness. And the more you practice mindfulness, the more relaxed and peaceful within yourself you become. In the words of Jon Kabat-Zinn, a respected leader in mindfulness meditation, "You are training your mind to be less reactive and more stable."

Natural Woman

Jon Kabat-Zinn, Ph.D., is the founder of the University of Massachusetts Center for Mindfulness in Medicine, Health Care, and Society at the University of Massachusetts Medical School. His mind-body integration and mindfulness meditation techniques are widely taught, both by Kabat-Zinn himself and by others trained in the methods. Writing with his wife, Myla Kabat-Zinn, he applied the concepts of mindfulness to parenting in *Everyday Blessings: The Inner Work of Mindful Parenting* (New York: Hyperion, 1997).

Life Lives in the Moment

You're always thinking, but *what* are you thinking right now, this very instant? For as busy as your mind is, it's not always focused on the present moment—on what's happening *right now*. You have a lot of distractions competing for your attention.

The foundation of mindfulness is to bring awareness to the moment—and to each moment as it unfolds. When you do so, you leave yourself very little to worry about or fear—the past has already happened, and the future does not yet exist. Fears live in the future, which does not exist and is highly unlikely to exist in the way we envision it. Worrying about the future means you miss what's happening in the here and now, and all that worry causes stress—not to mention all the joys you miss in those moments that slip by unnoticed. In the end, you may find yourself saying, "If I'd known that was all there was to it, I wouldn't have worried about it!"

What If ...

When it comes to birth, we certainly have no shortage of fears and worries about what will happen. Indeed, the medical approach to birth pivots around the two most fear-mongering words in our vernacular: *what if*. Unfortunately, *what if* can take over when it comes to birthing: *What if something goes wrong?*

We sometimes express it not as a question, even, but as a statement, so ingrained is our belief that *what if* can only be *not good*. Even before we hear what follows them, those two little words shift focus from the exuberance of bringing a new life into the world to worries and fears about events that exist only in speculation and imagination.

What happened to, "*What if everything goes right?*" So *what if* can become you having the most ideal birth experience ever, with a healthy, perfect baby and an incredible bonding with your partner. *What if* can be a powerful affirmation as well. *What if* lives in the future. If you're going to envision anything that has yet to unfold, it should be what you want to happen rather than what you fear.

Let's go back, then, to where we started in this chapter and do a retake—what do you look forward to the most about the birthing experience that lies ahead? Many things, we're sure; choose one for right now, and you can come back to the others later. Let this thought bubble rise. Don't be surprised if this is harder. Relax ... it'll come. Many of us tend to bury the good stuff much deeper—as much as we may fear that thinking about something that scares us will make that something happen, we conversely, and perversely, fear that thinking something good will make it not happen.

Go ahead and let your thoughts thoroughly explore and enjoy this anticipation. Do you have any of the judgments attached like those that shadow your fears? (Often, not so much.) Do you want to climb right into this thought bubble and have the experience right now? This is the birthing you can have!

Fear, Stress, and Cortisol

Cortisol is your body's main stress hormone. It puts out the call for help from adrenaline and noradrenaline, other hormones that are part of the stress response, to get your heart pounding and your muscles ready to haul out of there, even if there really isn't anything from which to flee. It's your flight-or-fight response, and it knows only those two options. And when your cortisol level goes up, your baby's cortisol level goes up, too. Much of what's happening in your body is also happening in your baby's body.

> **Oh, Baby!** _____
>
> Sustained exposure to higher-than-normal levels of cortisol leads to a host of health concerns in adults. We don't really know how such exposure affects an unborn baby, although we have to presume that it does have an effect. Some studies suggest excessive cortisol exposure before birth may slow a baby's early intellectual development, with the baby not catching up until age 18 months or older.

In the natural scheme of things, the stress hormones—cortisol, adrenaline, and noradrenaline—are essential for birthing. Cortisol helps set in motion the shift in balance between estrogen and progesterone that gets labor going, and it helps prepare your baby for its journey to the outside world. But cortisol turns against you when the amount of cortisol in your blood circulation becomes high and stays high; it begins to interfere with the normal birthing process.

Along with all the many other ways cortisol affects your body, it also blocks oxytocin—the hormone of love that releases those lovely endorphins for natural pain relief and also the hormone of action that keeps your uterus contracting as it should (Chapter 4 discusses the roles of hormones in birth). The primal way that hormones function is an effective check-and-balance system: if you're feeling relaxed and euphoric, as when oxytocin and endorphin levels are high and cortisol level is low, you're probably not going to feel like running or fighting! Meditation, yoga, and massage (which Chapter 10 discusses) are methods that help lower cortisol and raise oxytocin.

Mind over Matter

You can't think your way through labor and birthing. You have to give yourself over to the flow of forces, both within you and outside you, that are beyond your control. You can ride the waves of those forces, however, by allowing them to occupy your attention and awareness.

Focus on the breath, as in yoga breathing (see Chapter 10), is deeply calming and relaxing because nothing else matters but the object of your focus: your breath. Your emotions and feelings are still there; you're just not judging them or trying to control them. Your meditative focus puts them in a sort of suspended animation. In birthing, this focus releases your body so it can do what it wants and needs to do to birth your baby.

> **Natural Woman** _____
>
> Breath work—meditative focus on the breath and its movement in, through, and out of your body—is a way to stay centered, grounded, and relaxed within yourself so your body can do the work of birthing without interference from your conscious brain. When it is most effective, breath work can change what you feel during the birth and even take pain out of the equation. Instead, during birthing you might feel pressure, with big pressure right before crowning begins. You might feel your baby helping you, too, by pushing off your ribs until your baby is too low in your pelvis to make contact any more.

Mindfulness turns the focus on those feelings and thoughts. The concept is that when you can safely (nonjudgmentally) explore your emotions, you can allow them to exist for what they are without feeling the need to act upon them or let them influence you. Like transcendental approaches, this validates your emotions but removes their ability to affect you or scare you.

Mindfulness is often insightful because when you can examine thoughts and feelings without judging them, you often can see the outside factors that are driving them. These are the agendas and intentions of others, not of you, and they're making waves in your mind. Now, trying to stop waves is beyond futile, but you can ride them like you're on a surfboard. This is not really about control, but about deciding to go with the flow and letting go of the perceived need to *do something* about it. Your contractions will feel like big waves, and with each you'll know they are doing some work. With mindfulness, you can comment on that to yourself without getting into a thought process that spooks you into thinking about fear-based things. With birthing, it's easy to stray from what matters to *you* because sometimes other people—providers, friends, family members—may want you to feel and do what matters to *them*. You can find yourself caught up in outside pressures from people who want to impose their perspectives on you, and that can get tiresome really fast. Stay in the moment! Doing so will keep you focused on what truly matters.

Share the Moment

You can use mindfulness methods anywhere, any time, without any assistance from anyone else. That's part of their beauty—there are no restrictions. However, you don't have to go solo with them; you can involve your partner, your midwife, even your older children.

> **Trusty Midwife Tips**
>
> Once you become aware and mindful of the birthing experience, the motivations of others become clearer to you as well. You're able to see things for what they are and respond to them calmly and rationally, which helps you make choices and decisions without getting caught up in emotions—your own and those of others.

Many couples take mindfulness meditation classes together. Your partner can use mindfulness techniques to help him stay calm and focused so he can be there to support you as you need him to when things get intense. And because he knows the techniques you're using, he can help guide you and encourage you in your own mindfulness practices. Dads have their own anxieties, too, about what they should be doing or knowing at any given moment throughout the birth.

Beyond Birth

As the time for birthing approaches, it's natural to direct most of your thoughts and emotions there. But whether this is your first baby or you have a gaggle of siblings waiting to meet the newest addition to your family, your life will change with this baby's birth. Each baby only gets one birth. As much as you're looking forward to your baby's arrival, you may have worries and concerns about the changes the baby will create in your life and your lifestyle. It's normal to feel this way. Not very productive, but definitely normal.

The mindfulness methods you learn to use in labor and birthing are also helpful for calming these feelings. When your focus is on living in the moment, you can't be thinking about braces, first dates, first cars, and college. All those things are very far in the future and beyond your ability to control right now (and maybe then, too, but we won't go there …). So, take a breath, and fully experience the moment. When your mind wanders, explore the bubble and then go back to the breath, because that's where living is, right now.

Below the Surface of Consciousness: Calming the Energy

A number of approaches target energy rather than the physical body or the mind, although, of course, that's somewhat a matter of splitting hairs. As Albert Einstein most famously observed, everything is energy. Many *complementary therapies*, from acupuncture to yoga, are energy-based and are becoming increasingly popular in the United States, with about 40 percent of American adults using them in 2008. Most of these therapies have their origins in Eastern medicine (and in the United States, some in Native American medicine). In some other countries throughout the world, however, there's nothing complementary about these methods; they're part and parcel of the practice of medicine.

> **Birthing Book**
>
> Complementary therapies are treatment approaches that are outside the scope of conventional (allopathic) medicine. Complementary therapies are sometimes called alternative medicine.

As tends to be the case with energy methods and other complementary therapies, there's not a lot of empirical evidence—controlled, quantifiable studies—to substantiate their effects. (The exception is acupuncture, for which there are numerous studies supporting its effectiveness.) Many conventional physicians nonetheless are at least tolerant, if not supportive, of most complementary therapies on the premise that as long as they do no harm, they may do some good.

> **Oh, Baby!**
>
> Many of the methods used in natural birth are considered complementary or alternative by conventional medicine, including massage, breathing exercises, yoga, mindfulness and other forms of meditation, relaxation techniques, hypnosis, craniosacral therapy, visualization, and herbal remedies. Nonetheless, thousands of women have used (and do use) them and have found them highly effective.

In this chapter, we outline a few energy methods midwife Jenny believes can be beneficial—particularly acupressure. Other energy therapies that some women find helpful in pregnancy and during birthing include: craniosacral therapy (CST), reflexology, Reiki, and Total Body Modification (TBM). You may find that you get benefit from a good foot massage, for example, that's very much like the benefit you'd get from a reflexology treatment. The power of the energy within you is endless!

On Point: Acupressure

If you'd like to try acupuncture but aren't so keen on the needles, acupressure might be just the ticket for you. Acupressure is like acupuncture without the needles, using pressure instead. Acupressure beads (about the size of the point of a pen) on adhesive-backed pads are a common method for holding constant pressure against acupuncture points. Some acupressure beads are made of metal—gold, silver, copper, and blends. Many acupressure practitioners feel the metals do better at transmitting energy. Silver dampens down or decreases energy while gold elevates, activates, and increases. You can remain entirely mobile and even get into the shower or birthing tub with acupressure beads in place. You (or your partner) can also use your fingertips to apply pressure to, or to rub, acupuncture points.

Because acupuncture (the foundation of acupressure) is based on a network of energy pathways or meridians rather than anatomical structures, the acupressure points for certain effects may be quite distanced on your body from the area you want to affect. For example, pressure on the inside of your leg about four finger-widths up from your ankle bone (called the spleen 6 point) affects your cervix to initiate labor. Pressing firmly into the space between your thumb and forefinger, called the hoku point, affects your uterus. Rubbing the hoku point can give labor a jump start if it's going slowly or strengthen contractions when labor is well underway. Steady pressure on this point as a contraction is climbing to its peak can improve your comfort. There are charts online that show where these points are so you and your partner can learn to find them (just Google "acupressure points").

Acupuncture is highly effective for improved comfort during labor, too. The only drawback is that a qualified acupuncturist must insert the acupuncture needles, then remain present to monitor you because acupuncture can generate intense responses. Some midwives are also trained as acupuncturists, as are a smaller number of doctors. Like all things medical, however, licensing and practice requirements vary among states in the United States—and you know what this means: whether you can have acupuncture during birthing depends on where you live and whether the acupuncturist is willing to be on call for you and your birth.

Natural Woman _____

The cornerstone of traditional Chinese medicine (TCM), acupuncture is broadly practiced and accepted around the world—even as an anesthetic for surgery. Clinical studies support its effectiveness, especially to relieve dental pain, osteoarthritis, chronic low back pain, menstrual discomfort, addiction, depression, and anxiety. The Western perspective holds that acupuncture in some way activates the nervous system, which closely parallels the energy pathways in TCM.

Acupressure is also highly effective for relieving the nausea of morning sickness. Although morning sickness is common, affecting about half of pregnant women, no one knows for sure what causes it. Hormones most frequently get the blame, although certainly other factors are involved or every pregnant woman would experience it. There are three acupressure points for nausea:

◆ Pericardium 6 (PC6) is on the inside of your arm three finger-widths above your wrist. To locate it, lay your ring finger along the crease of your inner wrist and place your middle finger and forefinger alongside, like the Scout salute. PC 6 is on the thumb side of your inner arm where your forefinger rests.

◆ Kidney 27 (K27) is along the lower edge of your collarbone (clavicle), about two finger-widths from your breastbone (sternum), where there is a slight dip in the path of the bone.

◆ Kidney 6 (K6) is on the inside of your ankle at the small indentation in a bone called the medial malleus.

You can activate these points in several ways, and you may find that one works better than another for you. The first way is to apply firm, steady pressure yourself, with two fingers, when you're experiencing nausea. Hold the pressure for about five minutes. Obviously you can reach the acupressure point on only one side at a time with some points, so if you're still feeling queasy after five minutes, switch to apply pressure to the same point on the other side of your body.

You often get faster relief when someone else can apply pressure to the same set of points simultaneously—both K6 points, for example. And for extended relief, you can try Seabands and similar products, which are acupressure bands you wear over the PC6 points on your inner arms. The PC6 points are especially effective for motion sickness, and Seabands first came onto the market for this purpose. Make sure you apply pressure bands correctly (read the directions!) and wear them no longer than two hours at a time. The bands can be preventive, so you might want to put them on an hour or so before the time you usually feel nauseated if your morning sickness follows a predictable pattern.

Delving Deeper: Energy Methods

Other methods for relaxing the mind (and the body) are further removed from mainstream, although many women who choose natural birth use them. These methods fall collectively into the category of "energy work" and include craniosacral therapy (CST) (which is a favorite therapy of midwife Jenny's), Total Body Modification (TBM), Quantum Touch (QT), Therapeutic Touch (TT), Bach flower remedies, homeopathy, Qi Gong, and Reiki. As with acupuncture, these are methods that involve specific philosophies and procedures. If you're interested in trying any of them, it's important that you locate and use practitioners who are trained and certified in them. Some direct-entry midwives are trained in multiple complementary therapies, although nurse midwives and doctors seldom are.

Oh, Baby!

When having someone else activate acupressure points on your body, make sure to always do them in matching pairs. This maintains balance in the flow of energy and increases the effectiveness.

The underlying premise of energy methods is that blockages in the flow of energy occur that cause or contribute to a wide range of problems—emotional and physical tension, migraines, stress disorders, chronic pain and fatigue, and even orthopedic problems (especially those that affect the spine). As well, energy methods hold that the body, as the physical architecture of our human existence, further stores stress that manifests in physical signs such as hunched shoulders or perpetual worry. Energy methods may target the sites of physical signs or may address various energy channels (akin to acupuncture's premise of meridians).

Stay Tuned

No matter what methods you use, including ones that aren't "methods" at all but simply things that feel natural to you, a mindful birth is all about your awareness of your birthing experience. The more you know about all the many approaches to relax and open yourself fully to the work your body is doing to birth your baby, the better prepared you are to support those efforts. And that's what it's all about, right?

The Least You Need to Know

◆ Mindfulness allows your thoughts and emotions to exist without judgment or efforts to control them.

◆ Mindfulness and breathing techniques can help you relax and be comfortable throughout your pregnancy as well as during labor and birthing.

◆ Mindfulness techniques are helpful for partners, too, both for their own worries and concerns as well as for assisting the birthing woman.

◆ Energy methods are additional complementary ways to relieve stress, anxiety, and fear for a more comfortable birthing experience.

Chapter 12

Support for Going Natural

In This Chapter

- ◆ Choosing your support team and defining their roles
- ◆ Your team at a homebirth: tending to your comfort
- ◆ Your team at a birthing center: staging your environment
- ◆ Your team at a hospital birth: claiming your space
- ◆ What have you done today to make your dream birth become a reality?

This birth is all about you (and your baby, of course), although you have your best people ready to help you have your best birth, too. Your partner and midwife or doctor have key supporting roles. If you're planning a homebirth, perhaps you want to have your mother, sister, a friend, and other children there also. If you plan to birth in a birthing center or hospital, there are lots of other people whose jobs are to support you and your baby through labor, birthing, and immediate postpartum.

It's great to have all these people gathered around, but what are they going to *do*, actually? Well, ideally they'll do whatever you want. You're writer, director, and producer of this grand event, after all!

Now Playing: Your Birth!

The joy of pregnancy is contagious and can sometimes cause people to lose their sense of boundaries. Everyone wants to share in it, however fleetingly. Strangers waiting in the checkout line at the grocery store or riding in the elevator with you may launch into their own birth stories, offer advice on colic and temper tantrums, or even reach out to touch your belly without asking!

People get especially excited when a baby's birth time draws near. Family members and close friends may feel they should get to come to the birth, especially if it's to be a homebirth. Some might expect to receive hour-by-hour updates if it's to be a birthing center or hospital birth. It's easy, and sometimes fun, to get swept along in this enthusiasm yourself. Is it what you want, though? Birth is not a movie of the week, although it can take on that aura. It's a personal, private, and deeply intimate experience involving you, your baby, and your partner. Everyone else privileged enough to be present, including your health-care provider, is there to support you and to help you have your best birth experience.

So think carefully about who you want to invite to the birth and how they fit into the birth you envision. Will you be able to "go natural" in the truest sense—to let yourself go deep within yourself to that primal place where birth happens—when you have an audience? This isn't so easy for many women, even if they're people you love or they're gathered in another room.

Instead, there's a part of your brain that's struggling to think about what *they're* thinking, doing, or may need. To be true to yourself and to what's happening in your body, you need to feel fully safe to "go primal." Your support people should be thinking about what *you* need and making it happen for you before you need to ask. You have your mind on other things, and that's where it needs to stay.

The Home Team

When you choose to birth at home, you remain queen of the nest. No one comes or goes without your knowledge and approval. This is your place and your time; you're in charge. Your partner, midwife, and doula are all there to help you and to be sure everything goes the way you want it to happen. To make this scenario become a reality, you have to make sure everyone understands your vision and their roles in it.

Your partner can be a beacon of strength, support, love, and courage for you, as well as protector of your birth space, during labor and birth. Hopefully you're attending birthing preparation classes and preparing your birthing preferences together so your shared efforts are establishing a solid vision of the birth you desire. Many studies demonstrate the importance of loving touch during labor, including some smooching and snuggling to help you relax as well as to get that oxytocin flowing (more about this in Chapter 18).

Trusty Midwife Tips

Are there language or other issues, including vision or hearing impairment, for you or anyone on your support team? If so, include a person on your team who can translate for you or otherwise facilitate communication.

Trusty Midwife Tips

Is this birth an encore for you and your partner? It's still a good idea to take birthing classes. The methods you'll use during labor and birthing are most effective when you've practiced them so much that they've become second nature. What you don't use, you lose, as the saying goes—and even if you regularly practice methods such as meditation, you'll want to refresh yourself about applying them specifically in the context of birthing. Chapter 13 discusses birthing education.

Your Assignment Is ...

You may think that with a homebirth you can take things as they come, making the plan as you're going along. The opposite approach is more likely to result in your desired birth experience, however. Even if you're planning a homebirth, your written birthing preferences are crucial so when the birth is underway, everyone knows what to do and you're free to focus on what you're supposed to do, which is birth your baby.

Partners, family members, and friends sometimes become confused about what you want and how they can help during labor and birth, especially when the path of things isn't quite what they—and maybe you—expected. Giving each person specific assigned tasks and responsibilities takes the pressure off them trying to guess and also makes it more likely that you get everything you need.

> **Trusty Midwife Tips** _____
>
> Do you have other children at home? If so, include them in your planning and prep-aration. Even toddlers will be pleased to have special responsibilities to help get things ready for the new baby. If younger children will be staying with a friend or rela-tive while you're birthing, help them get their things ready. If older siblings will be present for the birth, you might consider taking them with you to one of your childbirth education classes (with permission from the instructor, of course) or at least sharing your thoughts and plans with them so they know what to expect.

Final Preparations

Although you're getting yourself ready for birth throughout your pregnancy, when the last month finally rolls around, it's time to get serious about preparations for homebirth. You're not packing a suitcase, but there are still things to do. Your partner can take care of details such as getting the birthing tub and making sure you have everything you need to hook it to your faucets (more about this in Chapter 14). You may feel like cooking, which is part of the nesting instinct. So put half of what you cook in the freezer so you'll have delicious, nutritious meals without any effort those first few weeks postpartum.

Reserve a drawer in your refrigerator for foods and drinks for when you're in labor, and let others in your household know this is your special stash. Lay in good supplies of your favorites, and make sure to include some special treats for yourself. Of course, fresh fruits and vegetables won't keep for long, so eat them while they're good. Just replace them and whatever else you might take from the "labor drawer" the same day. A shelf works for this purpose, too, although it's easier for other people to enjoy items that are simply on a shelf without realizing the snack is part of your labor stash.

Natural Birth in a Hospital

It's especially crucial for you to be in the driver's seat—the one in charge of where you're going and how you're getting there—if you choose a hospital for your birth. Not literally on the way there, of course; no one wants to be on the road with a woman in labor behind the wheel! But this is _your_ big event, and keeping the focus on what you want and expect will take persistent, consistent effort. Hopefully you've carefully chosen a provider and a hospital that support your intention for a natural birth (as Chapters 7 and 8 discuss), and you're discussing this intention with your provider at _each_ prenatal visit to help ingrain it with the provider, too. Every time you say the words "natural birth," your provider becomes that much more convinced you really mean what you say.

When your labor begins, it's natural to want to get to the hospital. You're excited, nervous, and eager to meet your baby. You may want to get there early so you can settle in and get comfortable before the real work of labor begins. Or you may be uncertain about how long things will take, especially if this is your first birth or you previously had a "fast" birth. But even your doctor or midwife will tell you: stay home as long as you can. We add: stay home even longer than you thought you would, because the longer you wait, the more likely it is that you'll get the birth experience you want. When you show up too early, there's plenty of time to "do" things, and odds are good they're not things you'd choose or that you may want.

At the hospital, a lot of people you've never met before are going to participate in your birthing experience. The presence of so many strangers in this most intimate and personal experience can be jarring. For a short time, you may feel that these strangers are closer to you than anyone in the world except maybe your partner—and then their shift ends and another round of strangers comes in. You can make this work for a natural birth; you just need to be prepared for it. The key is to always remember that this birth is yours, and how it unfolds is more important to you than it is to anyone else in the room.

Claim Your Space

It's a real mindset shift to treat a hospital room as your own space—your living room or bedroom. But it's a shift you have to make the moment you walk through the door. You need to make the space your own, right from the start, so you can feel like you belong rather than like a guest. Hospital staff already view this as *their* space, *their* routine, and *their* protocols. If you can keep this in the back of your mind, you'll be able to communicate more effectively to the staff that you want to personalize the energy of this birthing space as your own, and you'll be able to express what you want in a calm, measured way.

> **Trusty Midwife Tips**
>
> If you're birthing in a teaching hospital, your birth might be on the lesson plan for student nurses, midwives, and doctors. Although you're usually asked if this is okay with you (and you do have the option to decline), it's good to know in advance what to expect. Think about and discuss with your partner how you want to handle this. Birth is an intimate, glorious event and most providers remember with awe and delight the first birth in which they participated. But it is *your* birthing experience, so it's your decision.

You may be one birthing mom of many in a hospital staff day, but it is possible for the staff to see you as the unique woman you are and to relate to you one-on-one with respect for your experience. Claim your space as graciously as possible, and ask for nothing less.

Dealing with Protocols and Routines

Hospitals thrive on routines. Part of your learning curve now, before you're in the hospital, is to educate yourself about the routines that are in place at the hospital you're considering so you can decide in advance (your birthing preparations; see Chapter 17) which ones you'll accept and which ones you'll respectfully but firmly decline. It's good to discuss your preferences with your physician so you have the highest authority on your side—and better still, get your physician or provider to write your preferences into your admitting orders, especially if the hospital uses electronic medical records.

If your physician or provider disagrees with your preferences, what are the reasons? If you can't find common ground after talking through your respective views, it may be that these are not the right providers for you. Better to learn this now, when you still have time to make a change, than after you've checked into the hospital.

Having a natural birth in a hospital potentially means having to say "No thank you" or "Please, I'd like to" a lot. You'll want to do the research on your provider's policies so you can lay the groundwork for the staff's smooth acceptance of your requests. For example, you may want to say, "No, thanks, I'll wear my own clothes," because the first thing the hospital wants you to do when you check in is change into those nifty hospital jammies with the flapping back and tear-away sleeves. In a genuine emergency, whatever you're wearing is going to come off faster than you know, and if you don't care whether your own clothing gets soiled or bloody, why should they? You should wear whatever makes you comfortable. Or you may want to say, "I'd prefer the lights turned down low." Or "I've brought my favorite CDs to play."

It's okay for you to be the one with all the special requests and a million questions when such tenacity gets you your best birth. The support of your physician and provider is a crucial component of your birthing plan when you prepare for a natural birth in a hospital setting. Making your requests and asking your questions up front will make it a lot easier to anticipate and accommodate your desires when you arrive at the hospital in labor. For example, maybe you'd prefer not to have an IV started right away upon admittance; you'd like the opportunity to stay hydrated on your own, with your partner being sure that you're taking enough fluids. Under what circumstances would a physician and provider consider (and honor) this request?

Do a Doula

If you're birthing at a hospital, consider hiring an independent doula. You'll appreciate having a third party to watch out for your interests as well as to remind you of your birthing preferences—which sometimes get lost in the advice, suggestions, and intervention offers you'll be exposed to in a hospital setting. (Chapter 16 tells all about doulas.) A doula's not in love with you like your partner is, which is a very different filter to be watching you through during labor. A doula's not a midwife, either, so she's watching out only for your comfort. And an independent doula is not a hospital employee, so although she has to be mindful of hospital protocols, she's not bound to them.

An independent doula's sole objective is to help you have your best birth. Your doula can be the one who says, "No thanks" or "Please, she'd like to" and advocate on your behalf. A good doula keeps bent straws and fresh water in the water glasses, gets you up to pee even when you feel like you don't need to go, gives you a straw of honey or other nourishment, and turns off the lights so you can relax and sleep or focus. She also helps your partner support you and reminds hospital staff and others of your birthing preferences (see Chapter 17). Some doulas will come to your home when your labor begins and labor-sit with you. This is especially helpful if this is your first birth. An experienced doula can reassure you and let you know the best time for you to go to the hospital or whether it's truly too soon.

Oh, Baby!

Some hospitals do have doulas on staff who are available to any birthing woman who requests their services. However, it's important to recognize that a hospital-employed doula's first allegiance is to the hospital, and she may not be able to truly go the distance with you if you choose not to follow hospital protocols and procedures. Have a candid discussion with the doula about these issues early in your labor so you know how far you can go before you're out there by yourself.

An often underappreciated advantage to having a doula is that hospital staff tend to trust a doula's observations and opinions, particularly when the doula is often present at births in that hospital. The nurses know that although the doula is not a medical provider, she can recognize and alert them to anything that strays from normal.

> **Natural Woman**
>
> Some birthing centers allow you to come and go after you've checked in, so you can go out for a walk or even shopping if you choose. This gives a more relaxed, homelike feeling to the experience. You may be asked to stay within a certain time or distance range, though, so it's easy for you to return when your labor intensifies. If this interests you, ask about it when you interview birthing centers, or when you check in. You may need your provider to write an order.

Support in a Birthing Center

As Chapter 8 discusses, birthing centers can span the spectrum from being so home-like you'd love to move in, to being like a vacation hotel, to being difficult to distinguish from a hospital room. For a natural birth, you want to choose a birthing center that makes you feel like you could stay forever. Unlike the hospital, at a birthing center it's fine—and sometimes encouraged—for you to check in when your labor is still in its earlier stages. This gives you time to unpack, arrange your birthing space to suit you, and settle in. Your support team can settle themselves in, too.

Birthing centers usually don't have as many routine policies and procedures as hospitals, but they do have some. In arranging for your birth, you may have filled out documents to specify your preferences, which the staff will discuss with you in detail so everyone's on the same page when your labor gets underway. You also can expect an educational dialogue in response to your questions so you understand why the staff wants to do what they're proposing.

Some birthing centers have fully stocked kitchens so you don't have to worry about eating and drinking. Many women prefer to bring their own food, though, because it's what they're used to eating and packs no potential for unpleasant surprises (such as gastrointestinal upset) when you least want them. Most birthing centers have big showers and birthing tubs; some have Jacuzzi tubs. Your partner should bring swim wear to get in the water with you or stand with you in the shower.

Leave the Kitchen Sink; Bring Everything Else

When it comes time to pack the bags that will sit by the front door waiting for the time to go to the hospital or birthing center, you should collect everything you want to take—but your partner should pack it. That way, your partner knows where everything is and isn't going to ask in the middle of a contraction, "Honey, do you know where the address book is?" Then you'll have to stop your labor to say, "In the top right-hand pocket, under the flowered panties."

This is not good for your focus! It also helps your partner feel ownership about the birth bag and feel comfortable retrieving things from it, like your favorite pink slippers, without you first asking for them. If you need to take things with you that you still use every day, tape a note to the bag that lists those items and where they are. It can be like a little scavenger hunt for your partner to track them down and get them into the bag while you practice some relaxation techniques and make sure you're wearing matching shoes.

Remember that you're going to the hospital or birthing center to bring a baby home, not just because you're in labor. It's easy to lose sight of this. So take the car seat with you and also clothing for the baby to wear home. Bring a clean "going home" outfit for yourself, too—you won't want to come home in the same clothes you were wearing when you left, especially if you wore them during your labor. Your outfit should not be maternity clothes. Consider shopping for this outfit around your sixth or seventh month; what you buy then should easily and comfortably fit you postpartum.

Trusty Midwife Tips

When shopping for the outfit you'll be wearing home after your birth, think soft, comfy, and stretchy. Put your hand inside the clothing to gauge how it feels against your skin. After birth, your body remains in a heightened sense of physical awareness so what touches it may seem more intense. Clothing that has "give" is less likely to feel constraining or irritating.

All in the Family

Your family should be your strongest base of support. These are the people who love you, respect your choices and decisions, and will be integral in your new baby's life. How do they feel about natural birth? Sometimes you need to explain just what this means and that it's a safe alternative for birthing today. If any of your family members have had natural births themselves—a sister, perhaps—they already know the many benefits and joys of this experience. Perhaps they're why you've chosen to consider a natural birth for yourself. Supportive family members can provide encouragement and advice to help you in your own experiences.

Often, family members are eager to be part of your birthing. They may want to actually be present and have roles in the birth or be willing to take care of other children if you have them. They may sign on to cook, clean, and do your shopping for the weeks before and after the birth, freeing you to focus all your attention on your newest family member. When your family wants to be included, it's usually easy to find ways to do that to meet your needs and desires as well as theirs.

You can write your family members into your birthing preferences (see Chapter 17). This solidifies their importance in your birthing experience and also makes clear what you want (and don't want) them to do. It gives them identifiable tasks, which helps keep the peace and establish a sense of fairness. Everyone gets to share in the excitement of the new baby—and also in the chores and other activities important to keep the household running smoothly.

Your mother and your sisters may be especially important in your preparations for this birth. Your mother, of course, knows what it's like to give birth and manage the needs of a new baby in the family, no matter what the circumstances of her own birth experiences. Sisters share a special bond, and this is a good time to call on the connections you feel with your sisters. Any sisters who themselves have had births often can provide good advice.

Your family circle may also include grandparents, aunts and uncles, and cousins with whom you've maintained close relationships. In many families, the circle also includes dear friends who are "family by choice" and who will also likely enjoy and feel honored to be part of your birth.

Oh, Baby!

When you invite some family members and not others to your birthing, there may be hurt feelings. You can help mitigate this by asking those who won't be at the birth to have other kinds of participation in activities before and after the birth. Always remember that this is *your* birth, however, and try not to feel pressured to accommodate the wishes of others over your own wishes.

When Loved Ones Disagree

It's great when everyone important to you supports and encourages your choices and decisions about this birth. Sometimes, however, this isn't the case. You may encounter a range of reactions from confusion, disbelief, and even outright anger when you start telling people you're considering a natural birth. It can be difficult to try to balance everyone else's thoughts, ideas, and opinions with what you want for yourself, your baby, and your partner. It's often helpful to acknowledge that they disagree with you and also assure them that you're carefully researching natural birth as well as other birthing options (such as birthing centers) that may give you the birth experience you desire.

When it's your partner who disagrees with you, you have a bigger concern. You have to get to the bottom of the reasons why, and quickly, so you each can express your views and make shared decisions as parents. You may each need to decide what things are deal breakers—points you absolutely cannot give up—and what things you could negotiate to some point of middle ground. This is the stuff of parenting, too, so it's important to master the art of resolving your differences in ways that keep your baby's best interests at the center of your decisions.

Natural Woman

Your partner can be anyone you invite to have a primary role in your birthing experience. Relationships, pregnancy, and birth span a broad spectrum. "Family" encompasses not only those related to you by blood, but also the people with whom you choose to share your life experiences.

Asking for Support and Understanding

Birth is a big experience, and you'll need as much support as you can garner. Don't be afraid to ask friends, neighbors, and even coworkers for their help! Some people won't offer until you ask (and will be offended if you don't ask). You can draw upon these kinds of resources for a wide range of needs, from help with meals in the days before and after your birth to assistance with older children or even your pets. You won't know what people can and want to do until you offer them the opportunity to participate.

Nearly a Year to Practice

Your preparation goes on during your entire pregnancy, not just in the last few weeks when the reality of birth looms large. So, make sure every day that you consciously think about the birth you want and take at least one action toward making it a reality. Involve your partner and any other people who will be present at the birth, whether simply in conversation or in role-playing. There's no cheating in labor—and no do-overs or wait-a-minutes. What you don't address during your pregnancy, you'll end up addressing during labor—guaranteed.

When your birth team stays focused, it's easier to make informed decisions when choices arise. No decision *is* a decision! It's decision by default—and you don't want to default on your birth. No one can care more about what happens to you than you. Knowledge is power: knowledge of yourself, your partner, your provider, prenatal tests—and if you're going to the hospital, knowledge of the hospital and its procedures and protocols. You're about to have a life-altering experience, good or bad. You'll be the one who shapes it.

The Least You Need to Know

- You are the one in the driver's seat when it comes to getting your best birth.

- Discuss your birthing preferences with each person who will be present at the birth so everyone knows what you expect and what to do.

- Having a natural birth in a hospital means learning lots of ways to say "No thank you" or "Please, I'd prefer to."

- Have your partner pack your birth bag.

- No matter where your birth takes place, the most important function for your birth support team is to make sure the only thing that requires your attention is the birthing.

Part 4

Natural Birthing Methods

It's great to get your body and mind ready for birth, but you also need some specialized methods to improve your ability to focus and synchronize with your body's efforts—as if you were running a marathon. Breathing methods help you use your breath to relax your body and soothe your thoughts as well as to get plenty of oxygen into your system for you and your baby. Did you know being in a tub of water full enough that you can slightly float above the bottom takes away gravity—and pain? And hypnosis techniques help you stay calm, focused, and positive. The chapters in this part discuss these topics and more, giving you a full range of options for comfort without medication during labor and birth.

Chapter 3

Childbirth Preparation

In This Chapter

- Getting down to the details
- Read the (not so) fine print: is it education or preadmission?
- Modern Lamaze: go with your instincts
- Bradley: calm, quiet, and dark
- Mongan: no fear, no doubt

In some ways, it's counterintuitive to take classes to learn how to do something you already know, on a deep and primal level, how to do. However, birth preparation focuses on learning to *follow* your intuition and trust in your body's ability to birth. In this chapter, you learn the many methods you can use to work with your body's efforts and to open your thoughts and emotions to the joys of birthing.

Childbirth Education

For a long time, the focus in childbirth education was preparing for what can go wrong—the fear and doubt model. Finally, some approaches—notably Lamaze and Bradley (we talk about these later in this chapter)—boldly struck the position that (gasp!) women actually could birth without medication or intervention and (double gasp!) enjoy the experience.

The objective of any childbirth education program should be to provide women and their partners with information that encourages and supports them in their birthing decisions. However, this is not always the case. A lot of childbirth education classes range from "this is how our hospital functions" and a curriculum that looks more like it's for medical students to feel-good chat sessions with no curriculum whatsoever. It often takes some investigating to find the classes that fit your needs.

Run like the wind if the first session of your childbirth class presents birthing as a sequence of painful events for which there are modern methods to escape! No matter the kind of birth you intend, you want a joy-based, not fear-based, approach in your classes that presents birthing as the natural, wondrous experience it is. You can find such programs by talking with midwives, other women who have had natural births, and through online resources for methods that interest you. We discuss some of the common approaches later in this chapter, and the resources appendix at the end of this book provides additional information.

If you've already had at least one birth, you may want to find a refresher class. These are usually one-day events that present a summary of the topics you may have forgotten, that may have changed since your last birth, or are particularly important. Usually the same instructors or locations (such as hospitals and birthing centers) that teach the full course also offer the short course.

Trusty Midwife Tips

Most providers expect that you'll attend childbirth education classes of some sort. Many group practices—midwives and physicians alike—offer their own classes, which blend general preparation with specifics about how they do things. If you choose an independent childbirth education program, let your provider know so if there are handouts or forms you'd otherwise receive in their classes, you can get those.

Core Essentials

All childbirth education classes should cover certain core essentials about the birth experience. These include:

- What happens in your body as the time for birthing draws near and how to know when labor starts

- How to remain comfortable as labor progresses

- The progression of labor and how your baby moves through the birth path

◆ How specific events during labor may feel

◆ What methods you can use to assist your body's efforts while you stay calm and relaxed

◆ How your partner can support you and advocate for you

Most programs are structured for you to begin the classes when you're 30 to 32 weeks into your pregnancy. By then, not only have you realized this is for real, but you're also starting to think about the inevitability of birth. Your brain is ready to learn, and emotionally you're ready to practice. And most programs strongly encourage partners who will be at the birth to attend the classes; fee structures are usually for couples.

Some programs are precisely defined, and you get the same information presented in the same way whether you take the classes in San Francisco, Kansas City, or Boston. Others present kind of a free-form smorgasbord of methods that work well together, such as waterbirth, hypnosis (Chapters 13 and 14 cover these methods in detail), and breathing techniques. Others incorporate or adapt techniques from yoga, mindfulness meditation, and visualization specifically to labor and birth.

You may take a general class to learn about the process of birth, especially if this is your first birth, and then some classes in the specific methods that appeal to you. Online resources extend your access to all kinds of information, too. (See the resources appendix at the end of this book.)

> **Oh, Baby!**
>
> A lot of childbirth education classes include tours of a hospital birthing unit. If this is on the curriculum for the classes you're considering, it strongly suggests a medical orientation to the information the classes will present. Consider speaking with the instructor before you sign up, or ask if you can audit a class to see whether it's what you want.

Who's Teaching?

Most childbirth education instructors are trained and certified in the specific methods they teach and are often nurses or midwives. It's worth it to ask about the instructor's credentials, experience, and beliefs about birth. Sometimes hospital-based programs have a nurse from the labor and delivery unit teaching the classes, which is almost certainly a guarantee that the orientation is medical and information about natural birth is likely to be minimal.

As with providers, it's a good idea to ask for references—and to check them. Instructors who look great on paper may be boring, wander from the course outline, or have strident views on certain topics. Sometimes you can sit in on part of a class series currently underway and get a firsthand sense of the instructor's teaching ability, knowledge about the process of birth, and understanding of birthing options. If the class seems great but you can't understand (or stand) the instructor, find a different class. You won't go if you don't like the experience of it.

> **Trusty Midwife Tips** _____
>
> Birthing classes are most effective when you and your partner both attend. You get the same information at the same time, and can practice together with the guidance of the instructor. You and your partner bring different perspectives to the classes, as well, which can broaden and enhance your mutual understanding. Lastly, a birthing class is a safe environment in which to ask questions and express concerns—and others in the class may ask questions that haven't occurred to you or that you're reluctant to ask yourself.

If this is your first pregnancy, you might feel unsure about assessing the knowledge and ability of the instructor. Rely on your sensibility to guide you. Even if you're in the early stages of researching your birth options, you know more than you think. You have emotional reactions to what people say. If a birth educator is saying things that don't feel right to you, that's really all you need to know about that class—move on, it's not the class for you. Unless you're a birth practitioner yourself, you're not likely to have the same knowledge and understanding the instructor has. But you should be able to understand what the instructor says, in ways that make sense within your views and expectations surrounding birth.

Free at Your Local Hospital!

Ah, free is such a great price, isn't it? Well, as the saying goes, if it sounds too good to be true, it probably is. The classes may have no fees, but it's doubtful the birthing philosophy aligns with your desire to have a natural birth. Hospital birthing classes presume those attending are planning hospital births, as most are—and you may be, too, even as you're considering a natural birth.

But "free" here is really a sales pitch; the hospital is wooing you to come there for your birth. Sometimes you'll even get goodie bags with items such as coupons for meals in the hospital's cafeteria for waiting family and friends or a candlelight meal for two after your baby is born. Wouldn't you rather focus your attention on getting the birthing experience you want?

Not all hospitals offer free birthing classes. Many contract with outside consultants (nurses, midwives, and professional childbirth educators) to offer classes at the hospital campus. The consultant structures the class and usually charges a fee for participation. You're still likely to get a plug for the hospital, though, even when you pay for the class.

Approaches That Support Natural Birth

It's easy to think that all birthing education classes are pretty much the same, but nothing could be further from reality. As with providers, birthing classes tend to lean toward either a medical or a natural birth. Your first clue is the curriculum or syllabus (course outline): do you see sessions that present information about epidurals and c-sections? If you're intending a natural birth, these are not topics on your agenda! Does it hurt anything to learn about them? Probably not, although you may have to work to keep them in the perspective that matters to you. But when they're presented as the natural course of things, that tells you the class orientation is decidedly medical.

Some childbirth education programs are proprietary—they teach specific philosophies and techniques, and anyone who teaches them must complete training and receive certification from the program. With such programs, you usually have very small classes—sometimes only four to six couples, comprehensive materials, homework (yep!), and access to the instructor after the classes end for personal questions, reminders about how to do techniques, and other matters.

Birth Is Normal: The Lamaze Method

Firm in his belief that birth is a natural process, French obstetrician Fernand Lamaze (1891–1957) developed in the early 1950s the method of controlled breathing and other techniques that today bear his name. However, the modern practice of the Lamaze method looks little like its original design, which was modeled after Russian scientist Ivan Pavlov's *conditioned response* techniques most famously illustrated by dogs Pavlov conditioned to salivate at the sound of a bell. Pavlov's work was worthy of the Nobel Prize in Physiology or Medicine in 1904, and

> **Our Baby**
>
> **Birthing Book**
>
> **Conditioned response,** also called classical conditioning and associative learning, is a technique of gradually associating a stimulus with a desired response.

Lamaze's application of it in birthing became the first major success for women who wanted birth without medical intervention.

In the beginning, the Lamaze method was all about patterned breathing techniques to evoke a trained relaxation response with contractions during labor. Lamaze called the method psychoprophylaxis—prevention through use of the mind. He believed the breathing techniques also raised oxygen levels in the mother's blood, although this was later disproved. Lamaze also incorporated education about the birthing process so women fully understood what their bodies were doing. In an era in which twilight sleep was the hallmark of the birth experience for many women (see Chapter 1), the Lamaze method was a welcome breakthrough.

That was then; this is now. Gone are the patterned, practiced breathing and the heavy reliance on a birth coach. At the core of the Lamaze philosophy is the belief that birth is a normal process that requires no routine intervention of any kind. The modern Lamaze method emphasizes empowering women to follow their instincts to do what they already know: give birth. The 12 hours of Lamaze classes cover a wide range of topics for relaxation and comfort during labor and birth as well as information about breastfeeding and postpartum needs of both mother and baby.

Trusty Midwife Tips

Lamaze International is the organization that oversees the training and certification of Lamaze instructors as well as provides a wealth of resources and information for all levels of involvement with birthing. The website, www.lamaze.org, features resources, news, links to blogs, an online pregnancy newsletter, and a directory of certified Lamaze instructors. Look for LamazeOnline on Twitter (twitter.com), too.

Partners in Birthing: The Bradley Method

American obstetrician Robert Bradley, M.D. (1917–1998) developed the method that became today's 12-week course of instruction. It began in the 1950s with the goal of teaching fathers how to actively participate in the birth of their babies and how to coach their wives through birthing without drugs or anesthesia. It was a radical concept at its introduction—a time when fathers hung out in waiting rooms far removed from the birth. Bradley's hallmark analogy was to compare birthing to swimming and the role of the doctor to the role of the lifeguard. The doctor becomes necessary, like the lifeguard, only when problems develop.

Bradley's was also the first major voice advocating for calm, quiet, and near-darkness in the birthing place—and that's how births were when he was in attendance. He believed birth should proceed on its own timeline—another radical departure from his colleagues—and taught husbands to gently rub their wives' backs between contractions but to otherwise stay quiet. He taught women deep relaxation techniques, abdominal breathing methods, and physical conditioning exercises to help support their bodies in birthing. In a final break with the medical model, Bradley counseled women and their partners to themselves arrange the planning and circumstances for their births.

This partner/coach approach remains integral to the method today, although partners are not necessarily husbands. Of the 12 classes (which meet once a week for 12 weeks), two are dedicated to the role and functions of the birth coach. Often, Bradley Method instructors are themselves married couples. The Bradley Method also emphasizes maintaining good health throughout the pregnancy as an approach to keeping risk as low as possible.

> **Trusty Midwife Tips** _____
>
> The Bradley Method is the trademark of the American Academy of Husband-Coached Childbirth (AAHCC), founded by Dr. Robert Bradley in partnership with Jay and Marjie Hathaway. Only instructors trained and certified by the AAHCC are authorized to teach The Bradley Method. The AAHCC states that more than 86 percent of couples who use The Bradley Method have natural, nonmedicated births. Visit the website at www.bradleybirth.com to locate instructors in your area.

HypnoBirthing: The Mongan Method

Hypnotherapist Marie "Mickey" Mongan developed and began using her proprietary techniques for hypnosis to support natural birth in the early 1990s, the culmination of nearly four decades of study and interest in helping women experience birth without fear and doubt—allowing for comfortable, natural births. Today, HypnoBirthing, also called the Mongan Method, integrates education about the birthing process with techniques in relaxation, hypnosis, visualization, light touch, and techniques for "breathing the baby down" in birthing.

The curriculum is divided into five classes, each two and a half hours long. Instructors are trained and certified by HypnoBirthing International. The organization's website, www.hypnobirthing.com, features directories of practitioners who teach and use

HypnoBirthing (among them this book's coauthor/midwife Jenny) as well as providers and doulas who support HypnoBirthing. Chapter 14 discusses hypnosis in detail.

Preparation for Homebirth

If you're going to have a homebirth, do you still need childbirth education classes? We think so, as do most birth practitioners. Even if you've already had several births, there are always things you forget and advances that provide new ways of looking at things.

If you're considering homebirth, you've probably already found a midwife who does homebirths and will assist you. Odds are good that she teaches birthing education classes for her homebirth clients, or she may ask you to find your own classes from a list of local resources. She may focus on a specific method, such as HypnoBirthing, or combine a number of approaches that she has found work best. If there is a particular approach or technique that interests you, ask about it. There are lots of methods out there, and it's good to learn as much as you can about each one.

Oh, Baby!

Do you know the laws and regulations in your state that pertain to homebirth? You should! Ask your midwife to steer you toward resources on this topic so you can educate yourself. Although it's likely you'll never have to worry about state laws and regulations, it's wise to be aware of them!

Finding the Classes That Are Right for You

The best approach when it comes to childbirth education classes is to shop around as carefully as when you were choosing a provider. Feel free to call the instructors listed for the classes you want to take; they should enjoy talking with you to explain what they teach and why. If they don't, this also gives you useful information (run!).

Midwives, especially direct-entry midwives, are more likely than hospitals and doctors to recommend or offer classes that align with your birthing preferences and desires. But here, too, don't get shy about whether you feel there's a good fit between the two of you. Collect information and references, but in the end, you'll do best when you follow your intuition.

As with the search for the right provider, your quest for the right birthing classes can get confusing. Give your self a head start by first writing your thoughts about what you want to learn. If you know specifics, great; if not, you nonetheless probably have an idea of what you want to learn that draws from the kind of birthing experience you desire. Then collect information about the classes available in your area—where and how often they meet, who teaches them, how much they cost, and other information that may be relevant to your decision.

As you did in your provider search, ask other women what classes they took and what they thought of them. Ask the same questions of each woman you talk with, such as these:

- Did you look forward to going to each class?

- Did you understand what the instructor was teaching, and why the information was part of the class?

- Did the instructor accept and answer questions in each class?

- How did the instructor involve the class in active participation?

- Did you have any access to the instructor outside of class for questions not covered in class?

- Would you recommend this class to other pregnant women?

Always find out about details, such as policies for cancelled classes, missed classes, refunds, and extra expenses.

Not for Birthing Women Only!

Most birthing education programs assume your partner will participate with you in the methods you choose to use for comfort during labor and birthing. Most aim to empower you to take the lead; your partner is there not to coach you, which implies that your partner takes the lead, but to encourage and support you through whatever means make it so.

Having a doula somewhat takes your partner off the hook as far as being the one who rises to your defense when others challenge your choices and decisions. You might still need your partner to take on this role, but more importantly you need your partner to tell you that you're doing great, to rub that knotty spot in your lower back, and to repeat affirmations with you.

Trusty Midwife Tips _____

Are you planning to have your sister, mother, or dearest friend at your birth? Consider having her come with you to a birthing class. This provides a tangible framework for what you're learning and how you're viewing your birthing experience. Most classes will permit one "guest" visit, and nearly all will let you bring anyone you choose as long as you pay the fee for them. A guest visit to a birthing class is also a way to allay some of the concerns about natural birth.

If your partner has gone to all your birthing education classes, then the two of you have the same information from the same source. Your partner can use that information to help you in whatever ways you desire. The doula also can show the birth partner how or what to do and can stand in to let the partner take a break or nap.

The Least You Need to Know

◆ Many different childbirth education programs are available; some present specific philosophies and methods while others offer general information and a blend of approaches.

◆ Ask to see a full and detailed curriculum and the instructor's credentials, and meet the instructor before signing up for a childbirth education program.

◆ If your provider recommends a specific program or classes, ask for the reasons.

◆ Even if you've had previous births, a childbirth education refresher class is a good way to reconnect with what you know and perhaps learn new approaches or methods.

14

Waterbirth

In This Chapter

- ◆ Water reduces gravity by 75 percent
- ◆ Everyone—including you—will think you're too relaxed to be in labor
- ◆ What if your labor stops when you get in the water?
- ◆ Your baby's amazing dive reflex
- ◆ How to buy a birthing tub

Off the shore of the Hawaiian island of Kauai is an oddly shaped rock that looks somewhat like a chair. It has a short back and somewhat of a bowl in the seat, and the changing tides flow over it. This is the *Pohaku O Haoula*, the birthing stone of Hawaiian royalty in the fourteenth and fifteenth centuries. What a glorious experience that must have been, to float in the warm ocean water to birth your baby!

Although you can't go to the *Pohaku O Haoula* today except to admire it from the shore, what worked for ancient queens and princesses can work for you in the convenience of your birth location. A birthing tub can bring the concept and the comfort of waterbirth into your birthing experience.

Laboring Woman Defies Gravity!

What a headline that could be! Although at first you might think it rates right up there with "Woman Gives Birth to Three-Headed Alien Baby!", the best thing about it is that the story that follows is true.

"Upon entering the water, I let out a huge sigh of relief," said one of midwife Jenny's clients. "Another surge soon began, but I breathed through it easily. The relieving effect of the water was so great that I remember saying, 'Who needs an epidural when there's water?'"

Being in the water reduces the effect of gravity by as much as 75 percent. This is like walking on the moon, where the pull of gravity is so much less than on Earth that the astronauts who walked there during the Apollo missions in the late 1960s and early 1970s could easily bound more than 10 feet with each step.

> **Trusty Midwife Tips**
>
> The effect of water is so close to weightlessness that the U.S. National Aeronautics and Space Agency (NASA) uses pools for astronaut training. And on the flipside, scuba divers must attach weights to their bodies so they can remain underwater.

Gravity creates resistance, which in turn generates the need for effort to work against it. Hard-working muscles feel the pressure of their efforts, which can translate to discomfort and pain. Reducing the effect of gravity decreases the effort—so much so that you might think all you're doing is relaxing in the warm water. You can breathe the baby down, rather than pushing the baby down, and even catch your own baby. It's an astonishing and rewarding shift in the way you use your focus and your energy.

Many of midwife Jenny's clients have experiences similar to this one: "I reclined against the back of the tub a lot and would let my arms float freely in the water during surges. When I became uncomfortable, I moved freely and easily in the water to my newly adopted position. Midwife Jenny came to check on me, and I looked so calm and relaxed that she believed I was asleep and that my labor had stalled. But that was not the case, and shortly after the baby started to move down."

Less than an hour later, a new mother held her new daughter in her arms. "Words cannot describe the feelings experienced in that moment of time just following the birth," she said. "What a sense of empowerment, relief, joy, and overwhelming love!"

The Many Benefits of Water in Labor and Birthing

The force of gravity pulls on your uterus during contractions, putting a lot of pressure on your pelvic bones and other structures depending on your position. You may feel like each contraction is smashing you every which way. Being in the water allows everything to relax and open in any and every direction. Now there's less adrenaline because you're calm, and the birthing hormones can do their work. Labor becomes more effective and efficient.

In addition to significantly cutting the effect of gravity, water acts as "light touch" on the skin to release endorphins. Because these tactile sensations involve nearly your entire body all at once, the sense of relief and comfort you experience within seconds of getting into the birthing tub can feel dreamlike and surreal. Everywhere the water touches you, it causes the release of endorphins.

As you sit in the tub and gently float around in the water's buoyancy, it's like the water's giving you a continuous light-touch massage—and those endorphins just keep flowing. Your partner can enhance the effect by gently pouring warm water from the tub over your shoulders and back, if they're exposed above the surface of the water, or even across your belly if you're positioned in the tub such that it's poking up out of the water like a little island.

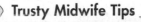

Trusty Midwife Tips

Water is especially beneficial for softening the perineal tissues, allowing them to more easily open for birthing. The comfort of the water also keeps you relaxed, which lessens the strain on all of the pink, perfect parts that are opening for the baby's passage.

About 70 percent of women who use birthing tubs during labor achieve their desire to have a natural, nonmedicated birth. When water is combined with methods such as hypnosis (which Chapter 15 discusses), mindfulness meditation, and other relaxation techniques, the likelihood for natural birth is even higher.

Wait a Minute ... Everything Has Stopped!

You may feel that you're so relaxed and calm in the birthing tub that your labor slows or even stops. Before you panic, however, just stand up for a couple minutes. If the grip of a strong contraction gives you a sudden reintroduction to the forces of gravity, you know the water has simply been doing its job—and lower yourself back into the water's warmth and comfort.

If you do stand out of the water for a few minutes (make sure to wrap a robe or blanket around you to stay warm) and feel nothing, then step out of the tub for 20 minutes or so. Some women produce an enzyme that causes labor, if it's not firmly established, to stop after they've been in the warm, soothing water for a while. Getting out of the water subdues this enzyme so labor can resume (and it will). When your contractions are again strong and regular, you can get back in the tub.

Some practitioners believe getting in the birthing tub in early labor causes labor to stop. Except for the few women who produce the enzyme discussed in the previous paragraph, this belief is not true. If your labor stops after you get in the tub, it was going to stop anyway. The solution is simple: your body needs a nap more than it needs to be in labor. Or you may need to walk around or do whatever you want to do. When your labor starts again, and it will, get back into the water. More often than not, however, getting into the birthing tub relaxes and calms you such that labor picks up—but you're so comfortable that you may not notice. There's little point in "saving" the tub for when labor gets serious. If you want to get in the tub, get in the tub. Trust your instincts!

> **Natural Woman**
>
> French physician Michel Odent, M.D., introduced birthing tubs into the mainstream of birthing practices in France in the 1970s. He then published the first article about waterbirth to appear in a peer-reviewed medical journal in the prestigious *Lancet* (1983). Dr. Odent's work has influenced birthing around the world.

There is a lingering and erroneous belief that gravity is necessary for birth to occur. This is no more true than the belief that a woman has to be squatting to get her pelvis to open enough to let a baby out. A *relaxed* birthing body works, period. Once you see and experience it, you'll readily believe it. And you have nothing to lose by giving it a try!

Birthing into Water

At first, the idea of birthing your baby into water sounds kind of scary. Won't the baby get water in his or her lungs when he or she tries to breathe? No. Prostaglandins, which are among the hormones that initiate the birthing process, rise in the baby's body and trigger changes in his lungs to help them prepare for breathing. Shortly before labor begins, the baby's lung movements—the "practice breathing" he's been doing for several months—cease. He's still receiving full oxygenation through the umbilical cord, which continues until he actually takes his first breaths of air.

If your baby is born underwater, the water does enter his throat (pharynx). But this activates a protective mechanism called the dive reflex that instantly closes access to the lungs. Although the baby may swallow water into his stomach, water can't get into his lungs. Blood flow continues to bring oxygen into his body. (The dive reflex remains until your baby is about six months old, which is why infants are such natural swimmers.)

When your baby surfaces, the change in pressure initiates a series of biochemical and physiological changes that cause him to begin breathing. Contact with the air on the baby's face sets in motion a series of changes that then switch the baby's oxygen supply to come from his lungs, and the blood flow from the placenta drops off.

Practitioners sometimes get nervous about waterbirth because they can't see what's going on under the water. But for a normal, natural birth, what's to see? Your midwife can feel to make sure the baby's not entangled in the umbilical cord in any way. If the cord is around the baby's neck or a limb, it's often easier to free it in the water. And you can check yourself to feel your progress, although you probably know without checking. But you can feel for the baby's position and certainly when the baby crowns.

Natural Woman

Recent research supports both the safety and effectiveness of waterbirth. Studies in Australia and England show that women who use waterbirth with their first pregnancies use less pain medication, have fewer perineal tears, and have a shorter pushing—as much as 90 minutes shorter.

If birthing your baby into the water makes you nervous, then don't! You can get out of the tub whenever you want, to have your baby in bed or where you choose. It may be challenging for you to move and also stay focused on your birth, but if you've alerted your midwife and your partner that you want to be out of the tub for the actual birth, they can be ready to help you. And they should be very ready to help, because changing from hydrostatic (water) pressure to atmospheric (air) pressure tends to shoot the baby out!

Who Should Avoid Waterbirth?

Waterbirth is appropriate for just about any birthing woman who has had a normal, low-risk pregnancy and is anticipating a normal, low-risk birth. What is sometimes a greater issue for women who want to use waterbirth is the availability of birthing tubs, especially in hospitals (more about that later in this chapter). If you are afraid of the water to the extent that you don't go swimming, you might find a birthing tub activates your fear because the water level is deep enough to let you float. However, the birthing tub's relatively small size and tall sides may help you feel contained and therefore more comfortable about being in the water.

Not Too Hot, Not Too Cold

It is important to maintain the water temperature within the recommended range—typically within two degrees either direction of normal body temperature. Generally, you don't want the water temperature lower than 97 degrees or higher than 102 degrees. Water that's too cold causes you to chill and shiver and can cause your baby to gasp when born, which will pull water into his lungs before his dive reflex activates.

Water that's too hot causes you to feel agitated and to sweat, even though you don't notice the sweating because you're already wet from being in the water, and can make the baby's heart rate go high and stay there. If the baby's heart rate does go up, it's a good sign to lower the temperature of the water and get out of the tub for a few minutes to let your body temperature go down. The baby's heart rate will return to normal, and you can get back into the slightly cooler water—and both of you will be just fine for the rest of the birth. Your midwife will be keeping tabs on both the water temperature and your baby's heart rate.

> **Trusty Midwife Tips**
>
> It takes 30 to 45 minutes to set up and fill most birthing tubs. It's good to coordinate with your partner and others who will be present at the birth so they know when to get started. Many women like to get the tub set up at the first signs of serious labor and fill it when they begin to feel the desire to be in the water. You can even climb into the tub as it is filling.

Birthing Tub Considerations

If you're considering a waterbirth, you'll want to get a special birthing tub (sometimes called a birthing pool). Most birthing tub designs feature soft, inflatable sides that are deep enough for the water to reach your armpits and large enough that your partner could get into the water with you if you want, but not so big that you could swim laps. You can set up a birthing tub anywhere, and there's access all the way around it.

Birthing tubs are fairly inexpensive to buy, from $40 to $300 or more. You can reuse the tub for future births or later use it as a soaking tub or as a kiddie pool (with only a small amount of water, of course). Some businesses rent birthing tubs, although the cost is often not much less than buying a tub. Using a liner with the tub makes cleanup easier.

When shopping for a tub (whether to buy or to rent), keep these factors in mind:

♦ **Is the tub deep enough?** You want the water to come nearly to your shoulders when you're sitting on the bottom. This water level will also cover your back if you get on your hands and knees but will easily allow you to keep your face and head out of the water.

♦ **Is the tub big enough for you to stretch out if you want or for your partner to get in with you?** If you're unsure, sit on the floor and stretch as you might if you were in the water, and have your partner measure. Compare this to the stated dimensions of the tubs you're considering.

♦ **Will your midwife be able to easily reach you from the side of the tub, no matter where you are in the tub?** It's possible for a birthing tub to be too big for you, too. If you can sit in the center of the tub and easily reach out to touch both sides at the same time, the tub size is probably about right.

♦ **Will the tub fit where you want to put it?** Measure out the size of the tub and see how much space it takes. This is especially an important consideration if you're planning to take your birthing tub to the hospital. It's a good idea to go to the hospital to measure and check out the faucet type so you have the right hardware to make the hose connections.

There are various styles of birthing tubs available, so don't feel you have to take the first thing you see. Make sure you order the filling kit and hoses; sometimes these are included in the cost of the tub, and sometimes they're extra. If you're having a tub shipped to you, it should arrive at least six weeks before the anticipated date of your birthing. *Be sure to do a trial setup long before labor begins.*

MacGyver Your Own Faucet Extension

Not all faucets will accept the filling kit adapter that comes with your birthing tub. Here's how to make your own faucet extension.

What you need: buy two or three inches of black rubber hose, such as for a washing machine, and two hose clamps. You'll also need the male end of a garden hose (the end with the threads on the outside), which you can buy from a hardware store or cut from a hose yourself. And you'll need a screwdriver (or a penny, if you really want to MacGyver all the way!) to tighten the hose clamps.

1. Clamp the metal male end of the hose onto the piece of black hose; you can do this beforehand. Make sure the second hose clamp is tight enough to stay on the hose until you need to use it. You will have to loosen it considerably once you are attaching it to the faucet itself.

2. Work the open end of the black hose over the outside of the faucet you want to use to fill the tub. Be sure to have the loosened second hose clamp on the black part of the hose *before* pushing the opposite end of the black hose over the faucet. You'll see that if you don't, you'll have to pull the black hose off the faucet and slide it on anyway.

3. Once you have enough black hose pushed up on the faucet end, slide the clamp up and make sure you have enough hose pushed up to accommodate the clamp and have it hold fast after the water pressure hits it when you turn on the faucet.

4. Now you can connect the faucet adapter that came with your tub to the male hose end to fill your tub.

Drain the tub when you're finished by activating the siphon mechanism on the adapter so the water runs down the drain. If you're not at home, be sure to take your black hose setup when you are finished draining the tub.

Will a Regular Bathtub Do?

Sure, nearly everyone has one. But regular bathtubs are not a very good option for waterbirth, although you certainly can sit in a bathtub of warm water just as you might stand in the shower. Most bathtubs are too narrow and short to let you move around, so you may not be comfortable being in the tub for very long. There's not much maneuvering room, either, and many women find it challenging first to seat themselves in the tub and then to stand up again when they want to get out of the tub. Bathtubs also have hard sides and are usually too shallow to fill deeply enough to cover you to your armpits. And they're usually built into a wall with only one side of the tub accessible.

Jacuzzi tubs, although deeper and larger, are also hard-sided and if built-in are not accessible from all sides. You may do fine to enjoy most of your labor in the Jacuzzi tub (especially if it has a heater that can keep the water temperature constant), although you may want or need to get out of the tub when it's time for the actual birth. Cleaning up after the birth becomes a different sort of consideration with a Jacuzzi tub, too.

Before birthing tubs became readily available, women who wanted waterbirth sometimes used inflatable kiddie pools. Though flexible and portable, the small size often isn't deep enough to fill with enough water to give you maximum comfort. Kiddie pools usually have brightly painted designs, too, which may be fun or annoying or distracting—although you could use a sheet or large towel as a liner to block them.

Trusty Midwife Tips

If you're planning a homebirth and want to use your regular bathtub for comfort during labor, consider placing a rubberized bath rug or mat, the kind you normally put on the floor outside the tub to drip on when you get out of the water, on the inside bottom of the tub. When you fill the tub with water the soft top surface will be more comfortable to sit on, and the rubberized backing will help keep the mat from slipping. For safety, have your partner or someone offer a steadying hand when you're getting in and out of the tub.

Running Water

A nice warm shower also helps relax tense muscles. Although you don't get the same gravity-defying effect of being suspended in the water, you do get an intensified "light massage" effect from the steady flow of water. You can take a chair or birthing ball into the shower to give some position options. Remember, though, that surfaces usually used when dry often become slippery when they get wet. It's a good idea to have a "spotter" close by—maybe your partner, doula, or midwife who can just sit in the room. Many women find the shower more comfortable and less confining than sitting in a regular bathtub.

Birthing Tubs and Hospitals

Although many birthing centers offer birthing tubs, hospitals haven't been quite so quick to embrace waterbirth. There are any number of reasons for this, but the deal-breaker seems to be the inability to effectively apply *universal precautions.* This is particularly an issue in the United States, where federal regulations as well as "best practices" standards establish the settings and procedures for following universal precautions.

Birthing Book

Universal precautions are the measures health-care providers take to protect themselves from contact with bodily fluids. Typical universal precautions include wearing gloves, protective clothing, and eye protection. In the United States, federal regulations establish the requirements for use of universal precautions.

Some hospitals will allow you to bring your own birthing tub. You'll probably have to sign a waiver that releases the hospital from any and all liability, but at least you can enjoy the benefits of being in the water. And the hospital may insist that you get out of the tub to actually birth your baby. You'll need to work out these kinds of details in advance with your provider and the hospital—and get the agreement in writing—so there are no unpleasant surprises when you want to set up your tub.

If you take your birthing tub to the hospital, also take lots of old beach towels that you can lay on the floor around the tub. Otherwise, you'll drip onto the vinyl flooring, making it slippery and cold. Your partner should bring swim wear to be able to get into the tub with you if you want that. It's also good to bring your own short stool so your partner can sit outside the tub and hold you or pour water on you. A chair will be too tall, and sitting or kneeling on the floor too short or uncomfortable; and kneeling won't last long on a hard floor.

Natural Woman

Have you had an injury to your tailbone? Such injuries are common and can be quite painful for a long time. Your baby's rotation against your tailbone can reactivate that pain. If you're in a birthing tub, two things happen to prevent that. One is that the water takes the pressure off your pelvis. The other is that you can easily move into positions that let your baby maneuver without pressing so tightly against your sacrum.

The Least You Need to Know

◆ Water deep enough to let your body float removes most of the effect of gravity.

◆ Standing in a shower is often more comfortable than sitting in a regular bathtub.

◆ It's air hitting a newborn's face, not the baby's emergence from your body, that activates the baby's breathing reflex.

◆ About 70 percent of women who use birthing tubs have natural, nonmedicated births.

Chapter 15

Birth with Hypnosis

In This Chapter

- ◆ Forget the stage shows!
- ◆ Hypnosis for anesthesia
- ◆ Daydreaming … or hypnosis "lite"?
- ◆ How to find a birth hypnotist
- ◆ Make the best of your positive beliefs

What if you could take the relaxation you feel with meditation, from a long massage, or upon waking after a good nap and extend it into a fully alert experience of calm and comfort during labor? You can—with hypnosis. About 70 percent of women who use hypnosis for birthing enjoy natural, nonmedicated births. More importantly, they have far fewer c-sections and an enjoyable labor and birth.

Hypnosis was the original "anesthesia" before doctors discovered the anesthetic properties of chemicals such as ether. Today, hypnosis is state-of-the-art, low-tech, and leading edge when it comes to relaxation and comfort in birthing. How can it be all that? Read on!

An Altered State of Attention

It's a great show on stages everywhere from the county fair to the glitter of Las Vegas. The hypnotist steps out and asks for volunteers, selecting maybe half a dozen from those who raise their hands. Some are shy, some do it on a dare, and some are boldly certain they'll turn the tables on the hypnotist by proving they can't be hypnotized. Minutes later, the entire group is singing and dancing—except the one who said he couldn't be hypnotized. That one's hopping around, flapping his arms and clucking like a demented chicken.

How is it possible for such a farce to have *any* therapeutic value, let alone have a role in natural birth? Well, first let's clear the air by saying there's nothing farcical, or even mystical, about hypnosis. And before we get too far ahead on the judgment curve, consider that clerks in shoe stores once used x-rays to fit shoes, too—even setting up x-ray machines in their store windows to entice the curious to come try this then-novelty (and of course to buy a new pair of shoes, perfectly fitted). We don't always understand the full scope and potential of new discoveries until they've been around for a while.

Hypnosis is simply a heightened state of attention, always available to you but seldom accessed. That's right—*heightened*. Did you think hypnosis was more like a deep sleep or a state of unconsciousness? Many people do, but the opposite is true. Indeed, stage hypnotists often tell their entertaining subjects that at the snap of fingers they'll "awaken" feeling as refreshed as if they'd had the best night's sleep ever. However, that's simply the reward (and not a bad one) to them for having danced around on the stage pretending to be rock stars or whatever other silliness the hypnotist chose to indulge for laughs. Although in an altered state of awareness, a hypnotized person is *fully awake* and *in control of his or her behavior*—even in stage shows.

Natural Woman _____

A woman using hypnosis in birthing often looks so calm and relaxed it doesn't seem possible that her body could be so intensely busy. Rather, she looks like she is, or is about to fall, asleep. The Greek origin of the word hypnosis, *hypnos*, in fact means sleep. But appearances are deceiving: she's very much awake, alert, and aware. She's just focused on shaping her experiences.

A Brief Hypnotic History

The first use of clinical hypnosis was as anesthesia for surgery. No carnival atmosphere here—this was the real deal, and the surgeries were often major. In the early 1900s, Russian doctors were using hypnosis in birthing women, often blending it with the breathing techniques being pioneered at the time by Fernand Lamaze. Lamaze breathing, being easier to teach and learn, soon took over—leaving the critical relaxation and fear release of hypnosis behind.

However, doctors trained in hypnosis continued to use the method for anesthesia in birth until the chemical anesthetics became popular in the 1930s. Although by and large ether and twilight sleep then displaced hypnosis, some advocates for natural birth, including British physician Dr. Grantly Dick-Read, persisted in using hypnotic techniques to help women relax and be comfortable during labor. And when interest in natural birth resurged in the 1970s, so did interest in hypnotic techniques.

Natural Woman

At the time when anesthetized childbirth was taking hold in Western countries, British obstetrician Grantly Dick-Read, M.D., (1890–1959) broke from convention and advocated for a shift in attitude to recognize and honor birth as the natural event that it was. Not surprisingly, the viewpoint was not very popular with Dick-Read's fellow physicians, who ostracized him. Dick-Read persisted, writing what would become the bible of the natural birth movement that is now in its fifth edition, *Childbirth without Fear: The Principles and Practice of Natural Childbirth* (first published in 1942 under the title *Revelation of Childbirth*).

What an Entrancing Experience!

The state of hypnosis is commonly called a trance because you don't look like you have more than a pinky finger in the waking world. Daydreaming, in which you take off in your mind on grand and glorious adventures, is like hypnosis-lite—a chance trance that just happens. You don't realize what you're doing or consciously direct the thoughts, images, and feelings in your mind (at least, at the onset). You sort of drift away. Once in the daydream, however, your conscious mind feels free to jump in to direct things, and if left uninterrupted you'll have quite the fantasy experience.

Unfortunately, in a chance trance there's usually someone or something that jolts you back to your surroundings. After recovering from the start, though, don't you feel relaxed and refreshed—like maybe you've really been away for a while? Another common experience of trance is pulling into the driveway and having no conscious memory of the drive home—your subconscious drove home for you. We've all experienced hypnosis—most often, though, not on purpose.

Oh, Baby! _____

There's a misperception that hypnosis somehow *creates* the birth experience you'll have. Hypnosis doesn't give you any particular birth experience, good or bad. Rather, hypnosis allows you to set aside your fears, worries, and beliefs about birthing so you can easily tap into your subconscious mind where the "inner you" knows how to birth with confidence and joy.

How Hypnosis Works

The short explanation of hypnosis is that no one knows for sure *how* it works! However, rather than being something done to you, hypnosis instead releases you to experience a natural state of awareness that *you* control and simply don't access most of the time. Although, you do drift in and out of an altered state when you become absorbed in a movie or a book, driving, or even simply your thoughts.

Some explain hypnosis as allowing the subconscious mind to "come out" and be in charge for a while. Because your subconscious mind doesn't know all the fears and worries you carry in your conscious mind, you have no expectations that they should affect the way you behave. Singing, dancing, and even hopping around acting like a chicken may seem silly behaviors on a stage—but are these silly behaviors, or do they appear silly because the people engaging in them are adults? Children play in these ways all the time because they have no learned experiences that have taught them how to think about these behaviors.

Trusty Midwife Tips _____

Combining hypnosis with waterbirth increases your likelihood of natural birth to about 90 percent. The water takes away gravity, which significantly relieves pain, pressure, and discomfort. The hypnosis helps you go deep within your subconscious mind to fully relax and concentrate your focus on flowing with the energy of your body. Women who combine these methods are often themselves amazed to realize the baby is well on its way along the birth path, or even crowning, and they have not experienced any of the classic markers of transition. In reality, of course, they have experienced them—just not in the way they were expecting.

There's also a dimension of hypnosis that seems to affect the brain's interpretation of nerve impulses. Signals that could be pain instead fade away. The brain also pumps up its production of endorphins, replacing any unpleasant interpretations with a wash of euphoria. As a relaxation and comfort technique in labor and birthing, hypnosis is self-induced; that is, you learn methods to put yourself into a hypnotic state, and you control how relaxed or how "deep" you want to go. No one can make you relax. Self-hypnosis is quite empowering because the woman has complete control of her decisions to use hypnotic techniques as well as the choices she makes during labor and birthing.

Believing Is Being

We all respond to suggestion, all the time—it's a hallmark of human nature. If it's 50 degrees outside and everyone in the office is talking about how cold it is, how likely are you to step outside and say, "Wow, it's really warm today!"? Not very—unless it's February and you're from Maine.

It's not that we can't think independently. It's that our brains process information through filters of perception that we create based on a blend of our own beliefs and expectations as well as those of other people. Hypnosis takes advantage of our susceptibility to suggestion by using it as a way to subdue the conscious mind's interference. Over time and with persistent repetition, suggestions become beliefs, and beliefs ultimately become behaviors.

> **Natural Woman**
>
> When you eliminate a negative belief, such as "birth has to hurt," something steps in to replace it. So why not intentionally replace it with a positive belief? For example, "my body and my baby know exactly what to do during birth." Then, the positive belief becomes what you dwell on, and it attracts further beliefs and behaviors that support it. Say and feel it, and you will create it.

Practice Makes Permanent

It's somewhat cliché but nonetheless true: what you practice is what you become. Some people believe—erroneously—that because hypnosis acts on the subconscious mind, there's nothing for the conscious mind to do. So they leave it all up to their class experiences, which works about as well as expecting to just close your eyes, open them, and be holding your baby. It doesn't work that way! Your conscious mind is used to and likes being in charge.

Most hypnosis methods for birthing include classes to teach techniques and homework to practice them, with CDs, scripts, affirmations, and other materials to help you stay focused. With practice and over time, you'll be able to engage and maintain a relaxed, hypnotic state for yourself at will. Many people like to continue using the hypnosis CDs or listen to certain music, however, because these act as suggestions to maintain attention in a specific way.

Control Issues

Some people worry that they won't be able to enter a hypnotic state because they're strong-willed and strong-minded—they not only like to be, but insist upon being, in control. Those who work with hypnosis say not only is that a myth, but people who are highly control-oriented are nearly always easier to hypnotize than people who say they're open to hypnosis. The reasons are complex, although likely distill down to the key factor in hypnosis: you are in control all the time. Someone who's really eager to try hypnosis may be expecting to cede control, which is not what happens.

When you use hypnotic techniques in labor and birthing, you're entering a hypnotic state on your own. At the beginning of your learning curve, the instructor will talk you into a state of relaxation so you can experience what it feels like. Sounds simple enough, doesn't it? Like any therapy, however, there's more to it than you think (and than we can cover here), but it is so simple because it is all up to you.

> **Trusty Midwife Tips**
>
> Is it just as good to learn hypnosis from a CD or videotapes? For many people, yes. The advantage of going to a "live" class or meeting with someone in person who teaches hypnosis methods is that the instructor can observe your efforts to use the methods and offer suggestions for improved success. Also, the instructor can hypnotize you, so you better know how it feels and what to expect.

Finding a Birth Hypnosis Program

The most direct route to explore hypnosis for birth is to take childbirth education classes that feature hypnosis as a primary technique for achieving relaxation and comfort during labor and birthing. The best known include the following.

◆ HypnoBirthing (also called the Mongan Method), developed by Marie "Mickey" Mongan, is a series of five classes with supportive materials. The parent organization provides training and certification for instructors, who then teach classes in their local areas. Chapter 13 gives an extended overview of HypnoBirthing (www.hypnobirthing.com), so we won't repeat it here.

◆ Hypnobabies (www.hypnobabies.com), developed by Kerry Tuschhoff, is a six-week series of classes that presents hypnosis from the orientation of its use as medical anesthesia based on the work of American hypnotherapist Gerald Kein. The parent organization trains and certifies instructors who then go forth to teach others. Hypnobabies also offers a home study program, using CDs to substitute for a live instructor along with all the materials of the regular classes, for those who can't find an instructor or do the classes in person.

◆ The Painless Childbirth Program (www.omnihypnosis.com), by respected clinical hypnotherapy instructor Gerald Kein, was one of the first hypnosis methods to become widely available for use in birthing. The Painless Childbirth Program is now only available on DVD; four DVDs provide nearly eight hours of comprehensive information and instruction.

◆ Natal Hypnotherapy (www.natalhypnotherapy.co.uk), developed by U.K. clinical hypnotherapist Maggie Howell, features classes presented over two days or four evenings. The parent organization trains its practitioners, who are then licensed to teach classes. There is also a CD version of the program, which currently is the only way to learn this method in the United States.

◆ New Way Childbirth (www.newwaychildbirth.com) is a home-study–only program of audio tapes and videotapes.

These methods have much in common, although they differ in philosophy and presentation. It's good to read about several approaches to understand how they're different. If you try one and it doesn't do much for you, change to another. Independently practicing hypnotherapists may also provide hypnosis for birthing. If you choose an independent hypnotherapist, ask how the program the hypnotherapist offers is specific for birthing and how much experience the hypnotherapist has in the birth room.

Instructor Qualifications

Instructors teaching specific birth hypnosis programs, such as HypnoBirthing or Hypnobabies, should show evidence of their certification if you ask to see it. The websites for the various programs contain lists of certified instructors, too, so you can double check. If the instructor does not have the appropriate certification, you don't really know what you're getting. She may be highly knowledgeable and qualified … or she may not. Because these programs follow structured curricula, you want a certified instructor.

> **Trusty Midwife Tips** _____
>
> Hypnotist, hypnotherapist—what's the difference? In a word, training. A hypnotist completes a specific course in hypnosis, although without a correlation to another field, such as psychology or sociology (counseling). A hypnotherapist completes a more extensive course of training that relates hypnotic techniques to counseling methods. The hypnosis techniques are the same, however, whether a hypnotist or hypnotherapist uses and teaches them. Often the only difference comes down to which is available in your local area.

Birth hypnosis instructors are not necessarily trained hypnotists or hypnotherapists, although some are. Nor are they necessarily certified childbirth educators … although some are. For hypnosis specific to birthing, what is important is that the instructor knows the methods of the birth hypnosis program. If you're going to learn hypnosis from an independent practitioner, it is important for that person to have appropriate training. The best way to assess this is to ask the practitioner and also to ask for and check with references. Ask to sit in on a class to see for yourself. Credentialing, licensing, certification, and even title (hypnotist or hypnotherapist) vary among states.

Partner Participation

Most birth hypnosis programs teach partners how to support the woman after she enters and maintains a hypnotic state as well as methods they may use to stay calm and focused, too. In some, the partner may have a role in helping the woman enter her hypnotic state during labor. A few hypnotists may prefer to train the partner to actually lead the woman into hypnosis. Many doulas are also trained in birth hypnosis and can also help guide the birthing woman into her blissful place. If you're going to use hypnosis and a doula, you'll need to find a doula who is trained in supporting a birth using hypnosis. The labor support is different; your doula can't "wing" it.

Is It Real?

There's some criticism that hypnosis is little more than a placebo effect; that is, it works because you believe it works. To a great extent, this is true, because hypnosis allows you to manifest your beliefs. When you believe you can experience a joyous, comfortable birth, all your efforts focus toward this outcome. Conversely, when you believe birth is inherently painful, it is. Hypnosis simply lets your conscious mind step out of the way so your beliefs can become your reality.

No matter the challenges to scientifically "prove" the effectiveness of hypnosis or to unravel how it works, one fact is incontrovertible: no harm comes to either mother or baby through the use of hypnotic techniques in birthing.

Trusty Midwife Tips

There have been some small studies in the last decade to evaluate the effectiveness of hypnosis in birthing, which suggest improved comfort and reduced need for pain relief medication. The findings were intriguing enough that now larger studies are underway—the most significant being one in the Australian state of Victoria that's looking at the experiences of thousands of women.

Surround Yourself with What You Want, Not What You Fear

Hypnosis gives you the opportunity to make the best of suggestions. Because comments of all kinds can influence your thoughts and beliefs, it makes good sense to keep yourself in the company of positive thinking. Letting people tell you only joyous stories of birth strengthens your knowledge that birth is joyous. You want to hear about methods for relaxation and comfort that worked.

Are you just putting your head in the sand with this approach, simply ignoring what you don't want to hear? No way! Why should you listen to all the negative, damaging things other people want to dump on you? No good reason that we know of. If someone starts down such a path with you, hold up your hand or gently interrupt. Say to the person, "Tell me about the best thing in your birthing." The both of you may be surprised by what follows.

The power of suggestion is strong even when you think you're blocking its effects, so keep yourself in a space where you can use what you hear to reinforce rather than defend what you believe about birth. In Chapter 2, we talked about the ways the words we use to describe birth influence our perceptions of the birthing experience. Through choosing the words you'll listen to, as well, you further shape and reinforce your confidence in your ability to have your best birthing experience.

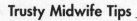

Trusty Midwife Tips _____

Overhearing conversations in hospitals is unfortunately common. Staff may stop outside your door to discuss someone else's condition, not thinking that you're right on the other side and able to hear just about as clearly as if you were standing beside them. Closed doors give the delusion of privacy. This is yet another reason to have music playing in your room. Some women even prefer to use headphones when they want to block out all distractions to focus on meditative techniques or their meditation CDs.

What you hear is particularly critical *during* the birthing when you're using hypnosis—because the filters of your conscious mind are bypassed, your subconscious mind takes everything as true while in a trance state. Overhearing doctors and nurses talking about another laboring woman's medical problems may easily enter your subconscious mind as a belief that you're the one having the problems. It's going to be hard to stay relaxed if you believe things are going badly and staff are keeping the information from you. There goes some adrenaline!

The Least You Need to Know

- ◆ Hypnosis is an altered state of awareness in which you are fully alert and in control; it is not a state of unconsciousness or deep sleep.

- ◆ Hypnotic techniques in labor and birth are self-induced; you use them yourself, and you control how deeply into a hypnotic state you go.

- ◆ When you're in a hypnotic state, you're highly susceptible to suggestions that are consistent with your beliefs; you will not do anything you do not want to do.

- ◆ In labor and birth, hypnotic methods allow you to deeply and fully relax to have the comfortable, joyful birthing experience you believe you can have.

16

Calling All Doulas

In This Chapter

- It really is Greek
- Birth and beyond
- One for me, one for you, and one for baby, too
- Choosing a doula

A doula can be the finishing touch for your best birthing experience. Her presence and participation can empower both you and your partner as well as leave you free to focus on the birth, each other, and your new baby. But what, exactly, is a doula ... besides an exotic-sounding word?

The word may be exotic, but the role that claims the title is about as down to earth as it gets. A doula is a personal support person whose sole responsibility is to look after you. Not in a birthing way; that's the role of your midwife or other practitioner. Not in a loving way; that's the role of your partner. Instead, in that way that's almost invisible—whatever you need is simply there for you. Sound a bit too good to be true? Relax! A doula is the real deal.

An Ancient Tradition

If you're thinking, "Huh, sounds Greek to me!", you're exactly right. The word *doula* has ancient origins—Greek, to be specific. The translation is somewhat vague, although in ancient times a doula was a woman of service, sometimes less than voluntary. But back in those times, servitude was one of the few "careers" available to ordinary women. A doula held special rank among the servants in a household—typically a household of wealth and social status.

Good doulas back in the days of ancient Greece were highly valued and cherished, as they are today, and often remained involved with a mother until the baby was two or three years old—through the breastfeeding period that was a young child's primary sustenance. With the prevailing belief being that early and frequent pregnancies and births were essential for a woman's health (to "open" her body so the "toxins" of menstruation could more freely flow), a good doula could have a lifetime position. Without such "relief" the woman would become poisoned, leading to an array of unpleasant interventions … but we won't go there.

Despite the modern aversion to the idea of servitude and even slavery associated with ancient doulas, the culture of that time revered and honored pregnancy and birth—albeit as a result of curious and peculiar beliefs, by our contemporary standards. Ancient physicians knew only what they could observe about the workings of the human body—and mostly their own bodies—which led to intriguing interpretations of bodily structures and functions.

A prevailing belief of the time (which persisted even into the eighteenth century) was that the uterus wandered about in a woman's body, making mischief and often illness. Most seriously, the wayward organ could perch atop the liver and cause a woman to have difficulty breathing or even suffocate—the liver being the organ of breathing in the ancient model of physiology. Only sex could lure the uterus to its proper place, and only pregnancy could tether it there. Hmm.

Custom, culture, and law did not permit women to be physicians (although a few were allowed to train as nurses to assist male physicians) and prohibited male physicians from examining women (which is why they needed female nurses to assist them). Midwives, who were more in number than physicians, tended births, although with only the knowledge and training acquired through experience. And doulas tended women in late pregnancy through labor, birth, and breastfeeding. In contemporary usage, "doula" has come to mean specifically "birthing assistant." Today, a doula is drawn to the role because she's committed to helping women experience their best and most joyous births.

Natural Woman _____

Only mere mortals had reason to turn to doulas for support and encouragement in labor and birthing. The mythic gods of ancient Greece birthed with fanfare suited to their status, as many myths tell. Aphrodite, the beautiful goddess of love and sex, rose from the foam of the sea. And Athena, the goddess of wisdom and war, burst from the head of her father, the god Zeus, fully grown and wearing armor. Another of Zeus's daughters, Artemis, goddess of the hunt and of childbirth, was born (along with twin Apollo) on a remote island after her father turned her mother into a small bird so she could give birth as easily as a bird lays an egg.

The Modern Doula

Today, doulas are popular and common throughout the world—no longer a service of privilege reserved for the wealthy and the social elite. Doulas support women in homebirth as well as birth in a hospital or birthing center and typically have strong working relationships with local birthing practitioners.

As with most practitioners who are outside the conventional medical model, qualifications and oversight vary widely. Some doulas still follow the "learn and earn" path of expertise through experience. Most doulas in the United States and many other countries attend training sessions and workshops to learn the fundamentals of pregnancy and birth as well as the many ways to support birthing women.

DONA International, the U.S.-based professional organization for doulas, cites a membership of more than 6,000 (most of which are in the United States). DONA International started its existence as Doulas of North America (the DONA part of the name), a modest effort to foster interest in doulas among both birthing women and women who wanted to be doulas. DONA offers a certification program intended to standardize the doula's role and level of knowledge. However, such certification is not mandatory.

Trusty Midwife Tips _____

Nearly all doulas today are women, although there are a few male doulas out there. In 2008 DONA reported that only 2 of its 6,000 members—who must be certified doulas—are men. Other men across the United States and Canada have completed doula training and may practice as doulas, though they have not sought certification.

Doulas, like midwives and physicians, have a wide range of philosophies and beliefs about birth. There's a tendency to presume all doulas, by virtue of their supportive roles, support and encourage natural birth. This is not true. Some doulas are very comfortable within the medical model and orient their supportive activities to be in alignment with medical birth. Other doulas are adamantly homebirth-oriented and never set foot inside hospitals … and only occasionally birthing centers.

The doula who is right for *you* is the doula who most closely matches your beliefs, birthing desires and preferences, and interests in comfort methods. If you're intending to use birth hypnosis and waterbirth, for example, you'll want to find a doula with experience working with women who use these approaches. A doula who has never seen, or is not a fan of, hypnosis isn't going to know *how* to support you and may wrongly panic at your calmness, thinking that you can't possibly be in labor and yet look like you're enjoying a very pleasant dream while you float in a birthing pool.

Conversely, a doula whose orientation is homebirth is not likely to be the support you need if you're planning a hospital birth. That said, some doulas are quite comfortable and experienced in accompanying you wherever you go in your birthing … from the birthing tub to the operating suite. You need to screen prospective doulas as carefully as you do for anyone who'll be with you during your birthing.

What Does a Doula Do?

A doula can do many things to help make your birthing experience more comfortable, from simply sitting with you to getting you blankets, keeping your water or juice glass fresh, reminding you (and others) of your birthing preferences if you get lost in the moment or seem to slide off track, reminding you and your partner to eat and sleep, and offering position changes if needed throughout the birth.

Trusty Midwife Tips

Not all doulas who have completed a DONA training program choose to become certified, because certification both defines and restricts what they're permitted to do. Some want to be free to do other functions, such as use a Doppler to check the baby's heart rate or be able to check on labor progress. These functions are outside the scope of a doula's certification; a person in this role is often called a *monitrice,* a term derived from French that loosely means "monitor."

Ideally, your birth partner is also right there with you from a loving perspective, guiding you through breathing, meditation, and/or affirmations. The efforts of the two of them—your partner and your doula—should flow seamlessly together to wrap a mantle of support and encouragement around you such that your focus can stay solely on the birthing. A doula does not replace your partner; rather, she supports you both.

Experienced doulas know much about the birthing centers and hospitals in their local areas. This is good, because one of the reasons you want a doula present is to know that when you need your doula to run interference for you, she knows how to take full advantage of the environment and personnel. A good doula knows which nurses support natural birth and which nurses are adamantly opposed—and how to push the envelope with policies and procedures without alienating staff.

Your doula cannot—and should not—make choices and decisions for you! Her role is to facilitate your birthing preferences to the best of her ability, not to define them for you. You and your partner still must take the lead and step in if the doula is struggling to get an idea, concept, or option across. It's also important to remember that a doula does not assist with birthing; she's a personal assistant for you, to meet all those needs that are indirect to the birthing but nonetheless essential for your comfort and confidence.

> **Oh, Baby!** _____
>
> A doula is not a midwife, although a midwife may act as a doula when she's not functioning as the birth attendant. A doula should not be involved in tasks related to birthing but rather is there to provide emotional support and tend to "creature comforts" to help you better focus on your birthing.

Birth Doula

A birth doula focuses on support for the mother primarily during labor and the birthing itself. She might come to your home to labor-sit with you in early labor, helping you to decide when is the appropriate time to leave for the birthing center or hospital if you've chosen one or the other for your birth location. If you're having a homebirth, your birth doula might help prepare the birthing tub, put clean sheets on your bed, make you soup and tea, walk with you—pretty much anything you'd like her to do to make you more comfortable. The idea is that the birth doula's activities free you to focus on the birthing.

When labor shifts and becomes more intense as birthing nears, your birth doula may do things such as adjust the lighting in the room, put the sign on the door that says "please enter gently," make sure the CDs or music that you want to listen to remain playing, bring you fresh bed linens or clothing if you're sweating a lot or moving in and out of the shower or birthing tub, place your slippers where you can easily slide into them, and keep cool, wet cloths ready for your partner to place against your fore-head or on the back of your neck.

A birth doula also pays close attention to what your midwife, or nurses and doctors, are doing and anticipates situations that may interrupt you (such as checking the baby's heart rate and your vital signs) so the interruptions are not so abrupt. Your birth doula should have read, and should have a copy of, your written birthing preferences.

Natural Woman

Most doulas offer at least one visit (some want two visits) prior to birth but may be available to you for weeks before your labor begins. You'll get at least one post-birth visit at home, maybe two, and have phone access throughout. Your doula should outline her services in a contract so everyone knows what is expected and what may be extra.

Your birth doula will usually stay with you for several hours after your birth, again focused on your comfort. She may bring you food and drink, help you get into clean, comfortable clothes, help you latch the baby on your breast, make sure you have plenty of pads, and if a homebirth, help your midwife clean up and put fresh sheets on the bed. When your midwife and doula leave after a homebirth, everything should be ready for you to use—clean, tidy, and inviting.

Postpartum Doula

A postpartum doula—who could be the same doula you had for birthing—sees to your comfort after the baby's born. She can guide you in caring for your new baby, if this is your first, and serve as a source of advice as well as assistance. Postpartum doulas usually have some training or expertise in breastfeeding, too, although they aren't lactation experts (more about breastfeeding in Chapter 21).

A postpartum doula also helps with routine household tasks including meal preparation for your family, cleaning up, and baby tasks such as diapering and bathing while you take a shower. If you have other children, a postpartum doula may teach them how to handle the new baby and instruct them in age-appropriate ways to help with the baby's care. You may use the services of a postpartum doula for a few days to a few weeks, depending on what you've negotiated with her.

Does Your Baby Need a Doula, Too?

Some people also hire a doula specifically for the baby to safeguard the baby's best interests with regard to the timing of clamping and cutting the umbilical cord or getting the baby right to the mom's chest following birth. A mother who does not have a birth partner may choose this approach, as might a couple who wants to so intimately share every moment of the birth experience with each other that they want only to remain immersed in the birth and welcoming their baby.

Whatever the circumstance, the mother doesn't want to have to think about the kinds of interruptions that may simply happen because they're standard procedures, such that they turn from looking deep into each other's eyes to find that their new baby is being whisked away for weighing, measuring, and other routine practices. A baby doula may also provide comfort measures for the baby, such as helping gently clean the baby when the mother's ready.

> **Trusty Midwife Tips** _____
>
> You might have a friend, neighbor, or even family member who offers to be your doula. Usually the person has birthed several children herself, and may serve as a doula for other people she knows. This arrangement can be a fine choice as long as you are both clear about the doula's role. You already know and trust each other. Although you may not feel comfortable writing up a contract (especially if you're not paying her), it's often helpful to sit down together and write a short list of what you each expect.

The doula you hire for yourself can also act as the baby doula. Just be clear in your birth preferences and at the time of contract signing that you expect your doula to protect the baby and your birthing space as well.

Doula Qualifications

There are no standard qualifications for someone to serve as a doula. Although most doulas do seek structured training and experience, some may take on the role simply based on their own experiences with birthing combined with a sense of satisfaction in being present at other births.

Hiring a Doula

Hiring a doula is much like the process you went through to choose your provider and birth location, and you can ask some of the same questions. In particular, you should ask:

♦ How do you feel about birth and pain? Make sure to have a detailed-enough conversation to determine whether she feels birth is inherently painful; this is not an orientation you want, whether or not you decide on a natural birth.

- Do you work alone? If so, what if it's a long birth—what do you do? And if not, how many other doulas are in your group? What happens if two births are happening at the same time?

- Have you been a doula for women who use hypnosis? Ask for specific examples.

Trusty Midwife Tips

Ask a prospective doula, "Do you believe birth has to be painful?" If she says yes or launches into an enormous monologue about why birth hurts, take a pass. As much as possible, you want to surround yourself with people who share *your* beliefs and expectations about birthing.

- What do you feel is your best role at a birth? (Some doulas will say, "To be as though I'm not even there" while others will launch into all they've done to "make" births happen. Doulas don't "make" births happen; this is a doula you want to avoid!)

- What would you do to help a woman whose labor is stalled or unexpectedly fast?

- Can you provide references of clients I can talk to? (Make sure, then, to get contact information so you can get in touch with the references.)

Meet the doula in person before agreeing to work with her, and either show her or talk to her about your birthing preferences. Pay attention to how she responds. Does she smile and nod but say nothing? Does she frown and say things like, "Well, in my experience …"? If she enthusiastically embraces your approach, does she talk about your birthing preferences with specifics from her experiences as a doula?

Oh, Baby!

Although a doula is not a medical professional, she is nonetheless bound by a code of ethics that guides her actions and behaviors. A key aspect of this is your right to privacy. If a doula that you're interviewing tosses around the names of her clients (especially any that are famous) during the conversation, keep looking. Your birthing experience is personal and intimate to you, and you need to be confident that others who share in it respect and honor this.

Trust your instincts. If for some reason a doula that you interview doesn't appeal to you, pay attention to that. Call at least three references. Be sure to have at least one, but probably more like two or three, pre-birth visits with the doula of your choice. This way, everybody knows ahead of time what the goals are and the most likely ways of achieving them.

Some doulas volunteer their services, although for most, doula-ing is a paying gig. Costs range from a few hundred to perhaps a thousand dollars, depending on the doula's services, the local market, and how much demand there is for the particular doula. However, a bigger price tag does not mean a better doula. Make sure you're clear on the doula's charges and payment procedures before you seal the deal.

An Independent Doula

When your doula works for herself, she works for you. There are no competing interests. No one else is writing her paychecks, so she doesn't have any confusion as far as knowing who she answers to. Your doula is there for you, period.

An independent doula may be part of a larger group or organization but does not work on salary for a hospital or a birthing center. This gives her the freedom to accept clients with whom she shares beliefs and expectations about birthing. Not every doula is right for every woman, just like any other service-oriented relationship. The doula your sister used and raved about for a full year following her birth may not appeal to you, or you might outright dislike each other. That's okay—you'll each move on, she to other clients and you to another doula. In most locations, there are plenty of choices.

> **Oh, Baby!** _____
> If you are considering a doula who works in a group so she has back-up coverage, be sure to meet all the doulas who may show up at your birth. If you are not comfortable with this kind of "call" arrangement, you'll probably want to find another doula.

A Staff Doula

Staff doulas work for hospitals and birthing centers. The intent of this is good and noble, and for many birthing women the available doula services are absolutely wonderful. Using a staff doula saves you the work of finding a reputable doula on your own; the hospital or birthing center has already verified qualifications, credentials, and the like—even run the obligatory police background check where required by law. You still pay for the doula's services, of course, but on your hospital or birthing center bill—and sometimes absorbed into it so you don't actually see a charge for doula services any more than you see one for nurse services.

You could run into a tricky situation when using a staff doula, however, if your birthing preferences include a strategy of informed refusal that challenges any of the facility's standard procedures. In this circumstance, a staff doula may not feel comfortable advocating on your behalf when it means she has to take on the organization that dispenses her paycheck. The situation can become one of an unfortunate tug-of-war between allegiances. This just means that you and your birth partner have to step up and relieve your doula from being "in the middle." Once the informed refusal is resolved, the doula can continue supporting you—or, if the refusal is more than the doula can accommodate for you, she can go home or move on to another birthing client in the hospital.

Collaborating for Your Best Birth

Many women who add a doula to their birth support team are grateful for the way things seem to simply happen when the doula's there. The doula is able to work in the background, freeing the woman and her partner to keep their attention solely on the process of birthing. As is always the case when the "background" works so smoothly, however, this kind of teamwork results from being clear about your expectations and from the doula being clear about her experience and the services she provides.

The Least You Need to Know

- A doula can provide emotional support and comfort-oriented services during labor, birth, and postpartum.

- A doula also can provide support in the weeks following birth, to help care for the baby and do light housekeeping tasks to take some of the load from you.

- Some doulas prefer homebirths, and others work exclusively with women who birth at birthing centers and hospitals.

- The best doula is one whose presence is barely noticeable.

Chapter 17

Making Your Birthing Preferences

In This Chapter

- What *do* you want?
- Write it long, write it short ... write it so it's right for you
- Dealing with deal breakers
- Nothing's carved in stone

You probably have a pretty good idea of what you want your birth experience to be like. If you've been following the suggestions in this book, you may have even envisioned your ideal birthing in such detail that it lives in your thoughts and emotions as though it has already happened. Now it's time to put the practical, tangible elements in place that can encourage and support your vision's reality.

Your birthing preferences help everyone else see what you see in your mind's eye. They put your dreams in writing. This gives the birth clarity for you as well as for everyone else who will participate in your birth, from your partner to your provider. Writing out your birthing preferences also helps you decide, in advance and removed from the heat of the moment, how you would like your provider to respond to any of the twists and turns that may occur during birth.

What You Prefer

Your vision for your birth defines your birthing preferences and the ideal birth as you envision it. It's crucial for you to hold this vision in your thoughts and emotions. However, no one can know how your birth will actually unfold. Some people talk about a birthing plan, and if you want to call it that, that's okay, too, as long as you can maintain flexibility. The challenge is that for most people, a plan implies a defined, even rigid structure that everyone follows no matter what. When there's a plan in place, we tend to lock onto it and expect it to take the path it lays out.

Birth's not like that. Birth follows its own script, and there are no previews to let us know, or even give us hints, how things will go. Of course it is important for you to have the most tangible vision of your birth as possible, but you can't cast in stone the path for your birth to follow. Rather, think of your birthing preferences as written in sand—they're there for all to see, yet everyone knows and accepts that they can change in a heartbeat.

> **Trusty Midwife Tips** _____
>
> Most birthing centers and many hospitals have birthing balls, birthing chairs, the ability to regulate the intensity of lighting in your birthing room, and other features to enhance your comfort during labor. If you want to bring your own accoutrements (especially a birthing tub), however, you may need to get this squared away ahead of time—possibly including permission in writing.

Put It in Writing

Your birthing preferences need to be in writing, and usually signed and dated, to carry any weight with providers and others who participate in your birth. The document you create then becomes part of the legal records of any provider and facility that receives a copy. This helps protect you as well as the provider or facility; you'll find that midwives, doctors, and nurses are all much more willing to honor your preferences when you've documented them in this way.

Your birthing preferences document can take any form that's comfortable for you. Some people write their preferences as though they're writing a letter. Others are quite didactic, listing possible events and their preferred actions or responses. Numerous online resources allow you to answer a series of questions and then generate a final "report" that summarizes your choices and responses. Here are some of the key issues to consider:

◆ If you desire a natural, nonmedicated labor and birth, make this the first thing you say: "I/we desire a natural, nonmedicated birth free from routine and unnecessary interruptions, procedures, and interventions."

◆ You may further define what you perceive such routine activities to be, specific to where you intend to have your birth: "I prefer to wear my own clothing, drink and eat my own food to remain hydrated and nourished, and allow my labor and birth to follow its natural progression and time frame."

◆ What are your provider's routine admission orders (standing orders)? Discuss their rationale with your provider, particularly those with which you disagree. Ask your provider to write specific admission orders for you that honor your preferences, such as for intermittent rather than continuous fetal monitoring, no admitting IV, permission to eat and drink, and no vaginal exams except by the provider.

◆ Who will be present during your labor and birth? Be specific: "I/we invite to our birth the following people …." You may further state, especially if you're intending a hospital birth, "I/we respectfully request that staff interruptions are minimal and no medical, nursing, or other students, or other observers, be present without our specific consent."

> **Trusty Midwife Tips**
>
> Are you keeping a memorabilia book for your baby? Consider putting a copy of your birthing preferences in it. It can be a touching record of the care and concern you put into crafting the best possible birth experience for your baby.

◆ Whose hands will receive the baby? They should be the hands of your partner or other person you choose for this honor, unless you're in the birthing tub or in a birthing position that lets you catch your baby yourself. Rarely in a normal, healthy birth is there any reason for the provider to be the one whose hands touch the baby first.

◆ What happens when the baby is born? You might say, "I desire for our baby to immediately be placed on my chest, skin-to-skin, with cord clamping delayed until the cord stops pulsing and after the placenta births, and for our baby to remain with me. We desire for our baby's father to then cut the cord. We request all routine measurements and such to be delayed for as long as the law permits, and for routine procedures to be done in our presence and preferably while one of us is holding or at least touching our baby."

◆ What happens in the hours following the birth? Specify that you want your baby with you at all times, that you're breastfeeding, and that you're caring for all of your baby's needs yourself.

Some concerns you may have should have already been worked out in the processes of choosing your provider and your birthing location (Chapters 7 and 8). For example, if you want a waterbirth, you should already know your provider supports this choice and the birthing center or hospital already provides a tub or will allow you to bring your own birthing tub. The facility should have written policies, procedures, or at a minimum, guidelines that make such matters clear. Many facilities have brochures that highlight their services from a marketing perspective, and then also provide you a written statement of their responsibilities, liabilities, and restrictions (you probably sign this with your preadmission paperwork).

Trusty Midwife Tips

Are you using hypnosis techniques for your labor and planning a hospital birth? If so, find out which nurses know about and support hypnosis, preferably on each shift. If possible, arrange to briefly meet them near the time of your birth. Then ask for one of these nurses when you check in. It never hurts to bring chocolate with you to share, too!

The facility likely has a checklist of preferred options, too, that you'll complete as part of your admission. It's a good idea to staple your birthing preferences document to this form so the two are always together. You'll also need several copies in your birth bag because you may have more than one nurse and more than one doctor as part of your birthing team.

Do keep in mind, however, that however carefully and thoroughly you prepare your birthing preferences, there is nothing legally or even ethically binding about them. They represent your desires and intentions, nothing else.

Say What You *Want* Your Birth Experience to Be

Every sentence in your birthing preferences needs to be about what you want, not what you don't want. You can look at this from the pragmatic perspective that what people read first is what they remember. So do you want that to be "natural birth" or "c-section"? You also can look at this from the perspective of the energy your words carry. What you focus on is what you're creating. Again, do you want that to be "natural birth" or "c-section"? Try it—read each of the following sentences out loud and see which sounds and feels better to you.

◆ We desire a natural birth, allowed to unfold in its own timing, in a calm and quiet setting, where we can welcome our baby with joy and love.

Or

◆ We do **NOT** want an epidural, an episiotomy, or a c-section unless an emergency arises that makes these interventions necessary to ensure the health of mother or baby.

And, of course, there's the tendency to add as much emphasis as possible on the **NOT** to make sure everyone gets that you don't want these things. The effect, however, is to make the most important word in the statement "not," followed by a list of all the nots. These "nots" become what the subconscious mind—yours and everyone else's—then incorporates as the anticipated experience, which of course is the exact opposite of your intention. You may think that both statements give the same message in the end, but really they don't. The first presumes a positive experience; the second presumes challenges and interventions. These presumptions shape the birthing experience both for you and for those who are with you, including your provider. If you're intending to have your birth in a hospital, the latter presumption is already in place in the mindset of staff—because hospitals function by being prepared for the worst and hoping for the best. It's a great mindset if you're having a heart attack, although not so much so for a normal, routine birth.

Further, the second statement presents a confrontational tone. You do want your birth preferences to set the stage that you're not the typical couple and that you're going to be doing something different. You want the staff on your side, to be partners and collaborators in helping you have your best birth. When your language and expectations are all positive, it helps staff to approach you in similar fashion—the premise that "like attracts like." What a difference presentation makes!

Trusty Midwife Tips

Most birthing centers and hospitals schedule a preadmission visit with you in the weeks before you expect to birth to take care of paperwork and routine matters. Even if you're told during this visit that what you've said in your birthing preferences is exactly how the facility does things, you'll still need to go over them with the nurses when you're actually admitted. The person who did your preadmission visit is not likely to be the one in your birthing suite.

Make Your Preferences as Long as You Need Them to Be

When you're planning a birthing center or hospital birth, you may find yourself thinking that brevity is more likely to get you what you want when it comes to stating your birthing preferences. (Sometimes the admitting guidelines will even suggest this.) Brevity is good when it serves your purpose, but there's no reason to be brief simply to make things easier for those who are reading your preferences.

Write as much as you need to clearly explain what you want (and sometimes to explain why). There's little value in keeping it short and sweet to make other people happy; this is your birth, remember! Those who participate should be striving to facilitate your best birth, not trying to fit you into their standard policies and procedures. If your birthing preferences document is more than one page in length, make sure the points that are the most important to you are on the first page. A lot of people, potentially, could be looking at your records, including your birthing preferences. Have someone stamp or label your birthing preferences document so it has all of your admitting information on it. Not only does this make the document look more official, it also makes it easy to verify that these are *your* preferences.

Who Gets a Copy?

Everyone who may participate in your birth should get a copy of your written birthing preferences, including you and your partner (you each should have your own copy). It's a good idea to have extra copies on hand, too, in case you end up with a substitution somewhere along the way. One prenatal appointment with your provider should be for the sole purpose of going over your preferences so you can discuss any differences of opinion and get them worked out in advance. Your provider should place a copy of your birthing preferences in your record and also include one with your admission orders.

If you go to a birthing center or hospital, give a copy of your preferences to the nurse who checks you in at admission. Does the nurse stop to read the document? Or does she set it aside and say it's already in your chart, or turn to her own preferences checklist? The ideal situation is that the nurse will stop to read it, make notes, discuss your preferences with you, and make more notes.

If the nurse disregards your birthing preferences document, you might be in for a time of reminding, reiterating, and defending. It's a good idea to give the nurse until the end of your admissions session to read and respond to your preferences; then if she doesn't, politely ask her to take a few minutes to go through them. It's important for the staff (which this nurse is representing) to know that you're serious about your preferences, you've put a lot of thought into them, and you intend to follow through on them as long as your birth remains normal.

> **Natural Woman** _____
>
> There isn't a doctor on the face of this earth who wouldn't understand a plea from a father saying, "She and I discussed this, and I'm telling you I'll have to sleep in the garage for the rest of my life if I don't do what we agreed."
>
> Everyone will chuckle and realize how hysterical and unreasonable a woman in labor can be (wink, wink) and how the partner is the voice of reason. Now, that's offensive on many levels—but in the heat of the moment, who cares? Sometimes you play whatever game that gets you what you want. You, too, can enjoy a laugh together about it when you're safely home with your baby and the birth story you share with others is the one you wanted to be able to tell.

Sometimes there's a nurse who does only admissions and who will tell you this. Here is the perfect opportunity to ask what nurses the admitting nurse would recommend to help you have the birthing experience you desire. The admitting nurse knows who's on the unit, who's on which shift, and who's most likely to support your birthing preferences—and can help pave the way toward your best birth.

Deal Breakers

Deal breakers are the things that you know you'll forever regret and resent about the birth. A deal breaker for you may be having an epidural, having your partner leave the room at any time, having the baby taken away for routine activities, having anyone other than the father receive the baby, or having anyone announce the sex of the baby to you—or all of these.

> **Oh, Baby!** _____
>
> Know what guidelines your provider and the facility where you intend to give birth follow for determining whether a c-section is necessary. When there are various decision points, specify in your birthing preferences that you desire to be fully informed and consulted about options and their pros and cons.

It's important for your partner to know your deal breakers and to be willing to step up for you. Sometimes this is hard, such as if you reach a point during your labor where you fling your natural birth intentions to the wind and insist on an epidural.

When you and your partner have discussed the potential for this situation to happen and have agreed on how your partner will handle it, your partner knows to remind you that you discussed this, what you're feeling is temporary, and you're only a short time away from holding your beautiful baby in your arms.

Well before the anticipated time of your birth, you and your partner should candidly and thoroughly discuss the possible scenarios that could challenge your deal breakers. You may even role-play them to make sure you each understand how the other views these scenarios. Labor's too late to discover you're not seeing things the same way.

Can You Change Your Mind?

In a word, yes. You can change your mind any time—about anything. Nothing's carved in stone; in fact, that's the point. We're talking preferences here, not rules or demands. This is all about what you want so that you can experience the birth you envision. You may indeed change your mind once labor begins; part of your discussions with your partner should include dialogue about what this would look like and how your partner knows you really mean it.

> **Trusty Midwife Tips**
>
> If you change your mind about something and feel you need to write this into your birthing preferences, do it as a separate document that says, "We make these changes to our original birthing preferences." Once you give copies of your birthing preferences to providers and facilities, they become part of your legal records and cannot be altered or replaced. You can only amend them. Put the change on the top so it's the first thing people read.

This can be tricky, because in the intensity of labor, you'll run the full gamut of emotions—and it's normal to hit some lows where you feel you just can't go on any longer. Your midwife can help you work through some of these kinds of concerns by telling you what she sees and how events usually work out, what's next, and what's normal.

Circumstances can change in quite literally a heartbeat, too. Your preferences address what you'd like your birthing experience to be, and often that's exactly what you get. But sometimes Mother Nature tosses a wild pitch and events take off in an unexpected direction. Always the most important factor must be the health of you and your baby.

Birthing preferences outline the ideal, although they also should acknowledge the possibility of the unexpected. If your baby takes an awkward position and an intervention becomes medically necessary, all things being equal (which sometimes doesn't happen), do you prefer a surgical vaginal intervention (such as episiotomy or vacuum extractor) or a c-section? It's important to be clear yourself and to have had this kind of discussion with both your partner and your provider.

Stay Flexible

It's the paradox of birth: you need to know, and be able to express, specifically what you want your birthing experience to be, yet at the same time you must be flexible enough to let go of those desires to go where the events of the birth take you as they unfold. All sorts of unexpected things can happen during birth—and many of them may be good things! When you're so focused on what you want to have happen, sometimes you miss what *is* happening.

Expect the Best!

This is a joyous time in your life, and you have every reason to expect your birthing experience to unfold just as you envision it. Stay focused on this vision, and on the positive, as you create your birthing preferences document. It's easy but unnecessary to slip into the "not" mode, and many templates for birthing preferences have just this kind of confrontational approach. Your birthing preferences should be about what you *do* want, which helps shape everyone else's perspective.

The Least You Need to Know

- ◆ Hold your best birth in your thoughts and visions, although remember that birth follows its own script and no one can know what will happen until it unfolds.

- ◆ Your attitude is the most important dimension of your birthing preferences and is the one factor you can for certain control.

- ◆ The more specific you are in crafting and expressing your birthing preferences, the more likely others participating in your birth are to collaborate with you to make them a reality.

- ◆ Give copies of your written birthing preferences to everyone who may participate in your birth, and discuss your preferences with the key players (your partner, midwife or doctor, doula, and the nurses if you go to a birthing center or hospital).

Part 5

Your Baby's Birthday Arrives!

You've read dozens of books, asked tons of questions, watched enough videos to feel like you actually know the people in them, talked with other moms who have had natural births, had countless late-night discussions with your partner—and when you look in the mirror, you can't see how your belly could possibly get any bigger. It's time. These chapters talk about what you can expect during labor, how to use what you've learned to keep yourself comfortable and relaxed, how your partner can share in the birth experience, and what to do when things don't quite go according to plan.

Chapter 18

Natural Labor

In This Chapter

- Just practicing
- Picking up the pace
- Okay, everybody … this is it!
- A transition so smooth and easy you didn't even notice

Movie melodrama would have you believe labor begins with a sudden, unmistakable, gripping contraction that stops you in your tracks. That may make everyone stop crunching their popcorn, but it's no more real than the butter on that popcorn.

In real life, you're more likely to feel some vague cramping and a bit of tightening—just enough that you wonder, "Is this it?" Then something distracts you, and when you return your attention to what you'd been feeling, it's gone. You don't always know it, but your body starts practicing as long as two weeks before the birth will occur. So how do you know when it's the real deal?

All the World's a Stage

Labor is your body's actions—hormonal, physical, emotional, and mental—to move your baby from your womb to your arms. You'd think labor is all about you—after all, it's your body that's making all the changes and doing all the work. But neither assumption is true. Although we don't know for certain what starts labor, scientists believe the baby's pituitary gland sends out the first hormonal signals that say, "Hey, I'm ready!" These signals set in motion the entire hormonal shift and the resulting changes in your body that cause labor to begin.

Your baby has quite a lot of work to do, as well. It's no stroll in the park to maneuver under that pubic arch and along the birth path. We don't know all of what happens in a baby's body to enable it to do all this adjusting and progressing, but we do know the baby is an active participant in birth. We also know that all those birthing hormones are helping your baby's lungs mature and setting into motion other physiologic changes so your baby's ready for that first breeze of air on her face.

> **Natural Woman**
>
> One of the most effective—and most enjoyable—ways to get labor going is sex. The prostaglandins in semen can stimulate the cervix, helping to nudge along the hormonal shifts that set labor in motion. A woman's orgasm releases a surge of oxytocin, which along with making her feel *really* good also causes the uterus to contract.

Labor progresses through three distinct stages. The timing of each—when it starts and how long it lasts—varies widely. Although generally speaking, labor is longer with a first birth than with subsequent births, there are plenty of first-time moms who know firsthand that this is certainly no hard-and-fast rule.

- Labor's first stage opens the cervix to allow the baby to pass through and occurs in three phases: early labor, active labor, and transition. The first stage of labor is the longest—what people commonly think of when they hear the word "labor"—and is the topic of this chapter.

- Labor's second stage is the descent of the baby to the outside world (and is the topic of Chapter 19).

- Labor's third stage is the birth of the placenta (also described in Chapter 19).

Women about to give birth mostly want to know whether what they're feeling is the real deal, so doctors, midwives, and just about everyone who notices your pregnancy all attempt to describe when and how labor starts. But the bottom line is that no one knows. Your labor may look a lot, a little, or nothing at all like anyone else's when it begins and even as it progresses.

Oh, Baby!

You may hear or read about "false labor"—contractions that really aren't contractions. But there's nothing false about them; they really happen, and you really feel them. It's much more appropriate to think of these episodes as practice labor, because those preliminary twinges and stretches are helping your body prepare for birth.

Dress Rehearsal: Prelabor

Prelabor is the beginning of your body's preparations for birth. You may think of it as warming up or like a dress rehearsal. It's not true labor, although it's a clear signal that the real thing is only days away. Prelabor can take many forms, and you may not experience all of them. Some women cruise through prelabor without recognizing that's what it is. Here are some of the common features of prelabor.

◆ **Nesting.** This burst of domesticity can take many appearances, from doing laundry, cleaning, cooking, and rearranging the living room at two in the morning to calling your partner at work because you need help switching the bedrooms around *right now*. Although the frenzy of your activities is often a source of amusement to others, it serves constructive purpose: you're getting everything set up so you don't have to deal with such tasks after your baby arrives.

Trusty Midwife Tips

A note to eager moms: fake nesting—running around doing all the things you might do during real nesting in an effort to cause labor to start—does not work. All you get are clean clothes, a spotless house, weeks of meals in the freezer, a new look in the living room, and not a contraction in sight. Your body will do what it's going to do when it's ready, and as the saying goes, you can't fool Mother Nature!

◆ **Practice labor.** You may experience episodes of uterine activity, cramps that feel like you're going to start your period, low back pain that nothing seems to relieve, and even some contractions that cause you to wake your partner and get out the watch with the second hand. But then it all fritters away after a few hours. This might disappoint you, but know that all these episodes of uterine activity *are* creating change. Your baby may drop a little lower, your cervix may open some or thin a bit, and you can practice your relaxation techniques. When it does come time for the labor that will bring your baby into your arms, it'll be shorter because you've already done some of the work in a fairly comfortable and convenient way.

♦ **Increase in vaginal discharge.** Sometimes you get a flood of vaginal discharge, fairly liquid, that's enough to make you think your bag of water has released, and you may need to wear a mini pad. This discharge is your body's natural lubricant to help your baby descend more easily during labor and birth, and it's likely to continue until birthing.

♦ **Feeling yucky.** You may wake up one morning and think maybe you've come down with something, so you call your midwife to say, "I think I'm sick." But when she questions you about symptoms—such as fever, headache, cough, nausea, vomiting, or diarrhea—it becomes clear you don't have anything. You just feel sick-ish. Your midwife may suggest you take it easy anyway because she knows you're not far from the start of labor. Your body's telling you that you need to sleep and rest, because in a day or two you'll be birthing your baby.

♦ **Zippity do-dah!** On the other hand, you may swing the opposite direction, bemusing your partner and calling your midwife to excitedly tell her you've been out shopping and now you're going to wallpaper and paint the kitchen. After a shared laugh and some chat about the colors and patterns you chose, you're likely to get the same gentle advice as if you had called to say how yucky you feel—take a nap and get some rest. This flood of energy could well be endorphins telling you your baby's nearly ready to come.

Early Labor

You may not know whether it's practice labor or early labor until it keeps going. And this is okay; it's easier on your nerves when you can ignore early labor. There's not much you or anyone can do, anyway, except wait for things to progress. Most early labor tends to be irregular and mild. You may feel like you want to sleep, which is good. Enjoy this opportunity, because it's going to be a while before you can sleep like this again! The old saying that a watched pot never boils is exceptionally true with early labor. So until your contractions really demand your full attention, just carry on with what you'd normally do. And having your water release in the grocery store usually gets you free groceries! There's no need to stay home "in case something happens."

Unplugged

You may lose your *mucus plug* in early labor. You may see it on your undies or floating in the toilet bowl—or you may not. It's not very conspicuous, looks more like snot than anything important, and usually you don't feel anything when it passes from your body. But its passing means your cervix is beginning to open, and that's a sure sign your labor's beginning. You may also have some blood show, which can range from a tint of pink on the toilet tissue to drops or threads of blood. This is further evidence that your cervix is in action. Or you may have no blood show, which is perfectly normal (and more likely when this is not your first baby).

> **Birthing Book**
>
> The **mucus plug** is a small, gluelike collection of cervical mucus and cells that forms in the cervix early in pregnancy and dislodges near the end of pregnancy when the cervix begins to change and soften in preparation for birth.

The Misperception of Breaking Water

It has become common "wisdom" that when your water breaks, you know you're in labor. Not exactly. Many women worry that their "water will break" and a flood of fluid will burst from them. It doesn't happen this way. The entire concept that anything breaks is a misnomer. As the baby drops into birthing position, the small section of the amniotic membranes that's in front of the baby's head bubbles out. Called the forebag, this bubble contains enough fluid to cushion the baby's head during contractions and to lubricate the birth path after the membranes tear ("rupture") as labor progresses. Many women never notice the release of fluid; others notice a trickle.

The forebag may rupture at *any* time during labor, letting the fluid out. This rupturing of the membranes occurs in about 98 percent of births. In the remaining 2 percent, the baby is born *en caul*; that is, with the amniotic sac intact around the baby. Most women have their membranes rupture late in labor, however, and the little gush of fluid that results helps to lubricate the baby's descent through the birth path.

> **Birthing Book**
>
> **En caul** is the term for a baby born enclosed within an intact amniotic sac. The birth attendant gently pulls the membranes from the baby's face at birth. In the folklore of many cultures, a baby born en caul is said to have special powers such as the ability to see mystic visions.

There have been a multitude of studies attempting to correlate the release of amniotic fluid before steady contractions begin with the presence of infection or some other problem. So far, there is no evidence for such a correlation. When your membranes spontaneously rupture, it simply means it's time to get down to the business of birthing your baby.

One of the methods commonly used as an attempt to get labor going is sweeping or stripping the membranes—a procedure that manipulates the contact between the membranes and the cervical os (interior opening of the cervix) that, while it does not actually rupture the membranes, disturbs the environment in ways that may nudge things along. If this is not effective, the next step is the artificial rupture of membranes (AROM). Sometimes this is effective for this purpose, and sometimes it's not—membrane rupture is only one of multiple factors that influence labor and must be aligned for labor to begin. It does have the effect of putting your labor "on the clock," however, because the medical perspective is that because the baby is now exposed to external bacteria, there's a risk for infection. The standard medical approach is to do whatever is necessary to birth the baby if labor doesn't result in birth within 24 hours.

There is a lot of anxiety around the potential for infection with membranes that rupture early in labor. Studies do support the 24-hour window; it takes at least that long for an infection to establish itself. Most women are strongly into labor by that time, because the baby's head is in direct application to the cervix and your body has only one response for this kind of pressure or stimulation: contractions to open the cervix. So it's very likely you'll be in active labor and birthing your baby well within the 24-hour window.

This Chair's Too Hard, It's Cold in Here, and Doesn't Anybody Know How to Make a Decent Sandwich?

Early labor could just as well be called the whiny stage, because nothing is right so you whine about it! You may not be so quick to pick up on this yourself, but if suddenly you're all alone because everyone has gone off to run errands or simply disappeared without saying anything to you, odds are good that you've hit the red zone on the whine-o-meter.

Women in early labor tend to feel edgy and out of sorts, although nothing in particular is wrong and they know it. It's different from the dip-or-zip feelings that characterize prelabor; there, you do feel like maybe you're sick, or conversely that you have superwoman energy. In this whiny phase, you're just restless. And you *know* you're restless, but you're unable to focus your energy and everything (including the people who love you and are trying to remain encouraging and upbeat) annoys you.

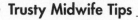

Trusty Midwife Tips _____

> If you're looking for something to do with your restless energy in the very early part of labor, think high tech. If you don't have one already, create a blog, or a Facebook or MySpace page—and if you do have one or more of these electronic presences, post to it. You could also set up your mass e-mail list for notifying everyone you know about the birth when it finally happens. And of course, you can tweet on Twitter.

The whiny stage does have a chatty flip side, so instead of whining and complaining you may instead move into chat mode. You find everything endlessly fascinating and worthy of discussion, from the color of the walls to the way the crust wraps so uniformly around a slice of bread. This, too, will pass—much to everyone's relief.

Put Up Your Feet, Take a Rest

You're excited to be in labor, so of course you want to get yourself to the location where you want to have your birth. You can settle in, arrange things to your satisfaction, and get this show ready to roll. If you're intending a homebirth, great—you're already there.

If you're planning to have your birth at a birthing center or hospital, go for a walk instead. If you go now, they'll either send you home or feel compelled to "do" something to hurry things along, and it's not likely to be something you want.

As well, too long in the hospital feeds fear and doubt in you, and that's the last thing you want. So stay home and stay comfy until you feel like you don't want to move—that's the time to go to the birthing center or the hospital if that's your plan.

Trusty Midwife Tips _____

> Even _you_ may be so excited when labor finally begins that you want to call _everyone_ to let them know. Resist that urge! This is not where your focus should be. Everyone you call is going to get excited and anxious, too, wanting you or your partner to give regular updates on your progress—or most likely, will call you every two hours. Instead, after the baby's born (and it's okay to keep that news to yourself for a while), have your partner call one person who then calls everybody else. Find out what time is okay to call this one person, and have it all set up well in advance so there's no confusion. Make sure the number is in your partner's cell phone so the call is quick and easy to make without involving you.

Honey, It's Time!

Early labor shifts to active labor when your hormonal cocktail revs into, "Okay, everybody, we're having a baby!" mode. Your endorphins are on the rise, which puts the whining (or the chatting) to rest. You may begin going inward, less concerned about what's going on around you or who's there. And you're likely to be now having predictable contractions, although they may be six or seven minutes apart. Your partner has slipped back into the room to watch you, trying not to be obvious about timing your contractions. You're into your relaxation and breathing techniques, and maybe the shower, so you're not really noticing anyway.

Natural Woman

If it's the middle of the night, it must be labor. At least that's the correlation for many mammals, including Rhesus monkeys—a species that has 99 percent the same genes as humans. Scientists speculate night birthing is so common because, in the primal world, the cover of darkness is protection.

A lot of providers, childbirth educators, and books say you should call when your contractions are about five minutes apart. However, your best marker for impending birth is not the clock but your focus and behavior. If you're still fussing about things or chatting away, you're pretty solidly in early labor. When it takes nearly all your concentration to ride the surge of a contraction, it's time for your partner to call your midwife, doctor, or hospital. *Now* you're having a baby.

Transition

Your contractions are going to get to about a minute apart as you approach active labor, which is very intense. You'll need all the support you can muster at this point— your full focus and concentration, all the methods you've learned and practiced, and all the encouragement your birthing team can give you. You're having another huge shift in your body's hormonal cocktail, and this is the one everyone's been waiting for. This is transition, the final phase of labor's first stage. You're almost there!

If you're in a bed or birthing chair, you might feel like you just can't do it anymore. You can't find a position that makes you comfortable. You have an almost irresistible urge to get out, get away, or go home if you're not there and anywhere else if you are. You may forget that this is the turning point, and you're going to have your baby soon. Instead, you may tell your partner and your provider you want *drugs* … anything that will relieve the pressure.

If you're in a birthing tub or using hypnosis techniques (and especially if you're using both), however, you may not experience these sensations and feelings in the same way. Instead, you're in that primal place deep within yourself where your body, thoughts, and emotions come together to give birth. You'll still feel pressure and your baby making progress, although you may feel like the surges are spacing out a bit—and they are, because your body is so deeply relaxed. You may even fall asleep between them, causing your partner to whisper to your midwife or doctor, "Is this normal?" It is!

 Natural Woman

According to the legend of the birth of Buddha, Buddha's mother Maya was walking near a grove of trees when she felt birth approaching. She stepped into the center of the trees and reached up to hold onto the branches of a sacred tree bending down to her. There, she gave birth while she was standing and felt no pain.

It's just not the common perception of transition, although it could (and should) be the common experience. Transition is designed to function as your body shifts from opening and thinning to the descent of the baby. Remember the hormonal loop from Chapter 4? This is the cycle of oxytocin to stimulate contractions and endorphins to relieve pain and establish a sense of euphoria, and it's in full swing by the time you reach transition. Even so, you might ask, how is it possible to fall asleep now, of all times, when you're right on the edge of giving birth? Well, what better time is there for a brief rest? Your body is wise, so it takes a break before the hormones shift.

Staying True to Your Best Birth

As labor intensifies, so does the attention you get from the nurses if you're birthing in a hospital. All their routines kick in; it's finally time for them to do what they do best. But that's not necessarily what you want them to do. This is also when your partner and your doula need to step up to diligently safeguard your birth. Hopefully you have everyone on the same page with you, including the nurses—and there's not much for anyone to do battle over once they realize this.

It's entirely possible that your labor may feel more intense to you but you're not showing any outward indications that it's actually progressing. This is normal when you've relocated from the comfort and familiarity of your home to a new and foreign environment. Leaving your house dumps adrenalin into your body, which slows or stops the oxytocin. This is like a pause button for your body.

Relax. Things will take off again. Have your partner or doula turn down the lights, politely shoo everyone else out, and put on your favorite CDs for music or for your hypnosis techniques. Get up, walk around, stand in the shower, or sit in a chair—whatever makes you feel most comfortable. Your contractions will return, sure and strong. Your body's doing just what it's supposed to do.

Trusty Midwife Tips

One of the most challenging aspects of early labor is going with the flow of your body. You of course have a lot of excitement because things are finally happening, and you want to keep them happening. You'll be much more comfortable and confident if you can let your body follow its own agenda in early labor, now and when the pace picks up. Practice labor and early labor are your opportunities to also practice becoming one with the process of birthing.

The Least You Need to Know

- Just about the only thing that's the same about labor for every woman is that it's the progression that births your baby; how this unfolds for you is uniquely your experience.

- Your behavior is a better marker for assessing how far along things are than are time or measures such as cervical opening and thinning.

- Although transition represents an intense effort on the part of your body, women who use methods such as water (birthing tub) and hypnosis often feel and appear so relaxed that a casual observer may not believe they're experiencing transition.

- Your labor will progress, even if you sometimes feel it's a process of one step forward and one step back; labor is a rhythm, not a stream.

Chapter 19

The Nonmedicated Birth

In This Chapter

◆ Finally ... it's time for a baby!

◆ Pushing works only when your body's ready to push

◆ Birth *really* is a big thing

◆ Let go of expectations, live in the moment

Much of the work of birthing is behind you as you reach labor's second stage and the purpose for all of this, your baby's birth. Now the focus shifts for everyone. You may be so totally in your primal place that no one else even exists in your awareness—only you and your baby, as it should be.

The goal with a nonmedicated birth is to be relaxed enough to tap into what your body already knows how to do, and to let it do that. This is a huge leap in listening to your inner wisdom and trusting yourself. Is it the leap for you? You might not know until you go for it.

"I Can't Do This Any Longer!"

"I can't do this any longer" is a universal pronouncement in labor, telling everyone that your baby is ready to be born. Nearly universal, too, is the sudden desire for an epidural if you've been at all uncertain about your ability to have a nonmedicated birth—your conscious brain knows this option is out there (although by this time it's usually too late for this). Fortunately, your body's one step ahead of your conscious brain and even as the words are coming out of your mouth your body has already responded with a jolt of adrenaline to energize you, accompanied by a flood of endorphins for that oh so lovely rush of euphoria that will herald the next phase of birth, down and out and into your arms.

It's a potent, irresistible combination that immediately refocuses and revitalizes you, which is especially welcome if you've had a long active phase of labor, and sends you back into your subconscious brain. You feel the strong urge to get yourself more upright to help your baby get into position for its final descent. You go deep within yourself again, so deep that nothing outside even exists for you. Sweat breaks out on your upper lip and it takes all your effort simply to focus on your breathing. You don't want anyone to touch you or talk to you, but you don't want your partner, midwife, and doula to leave. When you feel sure you can't do this anymore, crowning is imminent and then the drive to push comes from within and is impossible to ignore.

Sometimes you feel as if your labor's on the clock when you reach 10 centimeters. People might be telling you to push but all you can do is bear down, which isn't the same thing and causes you to hold your breath. And guess what? This bearing down hurts! There's no point in pushing when your body's not ready for you to push; it doesn't make things happen any faster.

If you're using hypnosis or you're in the birthing tub, or both, you often can breathe your baby all the way down to the perineum without any strong urges to push, though you will feel the urge to breathe down, grunt, or bear down. There should be no purple-faced breath-holding; when you're relaxed, you push with your body rather than at the command of someone else. The longest a woman will instinctively push is three to six seconds with breathing in between. This is how you get a 10-minute (or less!) pushing stage.

Trusty Midwife Tips

Midwife Jenny often has women in labor look up from the birthing tub and say to her shortly before birth is imminent, "This isn't fun anymore." It's an amazing shift in perspective, to be so enjoying labor that you consider it to be fun! Then comes the final stretch and you're tired because even when the experience is so good you don't want to stop, you just can't keep it going forever. Gotta love it!

Tuning in to Your Inner Messages

There's a constant inner dialogue going on during labor, no matter what methods you're using to focus and remain comfortable. You're very into yourself at this point, and might even be talking to yourself out loud. Much of what you say may sound nonsensical to others in the room, more like incoherent muttering or groaning. But to you it all makes perfect sense. Maybe you're instructing yourself to stay focused, repeating your vision of the birth you want to experience, saying affirmations, or even singing a favorite song. No matter what you're saying, you're also listening. You're fully engaged in this self-conversation, as though you've never before heard anything like it.

Mostly, this is really good because it keeps your attention focused on what's happening in your body rather than on the clock or on the other people in the room. However, it's important to listen also to the people outside you who are there to support and encourage you, especially if you're starting to think that things are not going right or that you can't do this. You chose these people to be with you for your birthing; now is the time to listen to them so they can be the help you want them to be. It's easy in your inner dialogue to overlook the tremendous progress, strength, and courage you're putting into your efforts and to instead talk yourself into "I can't." The key message you should hear from your birth support people is, "I'm so proud of you!" Because you are doing it, and doing it so very well.

The Essence of Time

Everyone worries about time when it comes to birth: when will labor start, how long will this phase last, how long will you feel like this, how long do the contractions last and how long is it between them, how long to push, when will the baby finally be born? Birth is more about timing than time; birth follows its own schedule. When labor is left alone and a woman feels comfortable and in control, it usually doesn't take longer than a day, start to finish, to birth a baby. Often it can take only six or eight hours.

Trusty Midwife Tips

One indication that the final efforts of birthing are underway is that you lose your awareness of time. You may think hours have gone by when it's been only minutes, or that it's been only minutes but it's really been several hours. This is good! Time, as the clock measures it, is an external construct. For you to be completely in the moment of your birthing experience, the only time that matters is that which your body is orchestrating.

Birthing exists very much in the moment. Every contraction is brand new; the one you just had is gone, and the one ahead of you hasn't happened yet. This can set up a sense of timelessness within you, if you're tuned into your body. When you're in that place where time does not exist, there's no pressure to meet any kind of timeline.

There truly is no "clock time" for how long you spend in each stage of labor, though this probably is not what you want to hear. Some women, at 3 or 4 centimeters, feel the need to set up the birthing tub or go to the hospital. Others want to take a nap. The defining question is: is the baby any lower? The answer tells much more about where you are along the arc of labor than does the measuring of dilation or the timing of contractions. How dilated you are doesn't tell anything about when your baby's going to arrive.

Trusty Midwife Tips

True transition is not 8 to 10 centimeters but is that lull before the storm. Everything you feel is "I gotta" and you cannot resist what your body wants to do. There's no reason to have a two-hour pushing phase; if you listen to your body, you can have that 10-minute pushing phase. When you feel that "baby in my butt" sensation, it's time to push in the next surge or two. You'll know. If you're not feeling this, then no one should be yelling at you to push because the baby's not yet low enough. Pushing now is a huge waste of energy and time with no gains.

"I'll Save That Until I *Really* Need It"

We're creatures of habit, and our habits have taught us to wait and save. We wait until we've eaten all the peas before we eat the ice cream. We save money to buy things or go places. And when it comes time for birth, we wait for labor to reach a certain measure (sometimes an arbitrary one) before calling the midwife, doctor, or hospital. We go into relaxation techniques to save energy for later, when we'll really need it. We wait to push. We "save" the birthing pool for when labor's going to be really hard.

We're well trained in this wait-and-save dynamic. However, you can begin using any and all of the methods you've learned and practiced—breathing techniques, yoga, meditation, massage, visualization, hypnosis, water—at any time during your labor. You won't slow, delay, or stop labor with any of the methods you've learned, no matter when or for how long you use them. Indeed, you might actually encourage things to accelerate because there's no anxiety in your body to create tension. Relaxation is the key. And if your labor does take a break, it's because you need a rest—even near the end, when it seems the pace should be picking up rather than tapping the pause button. Your labor will start again when your body's ready to resume its efforts.

Trusty Midwife Tips _____

When you've decided on a natural, nonmedicated birth, you need to remain calm enough to ask "why?" when people start making suggestions about medications (pain relief or labor stimulation) and other interventions. What, and how, do you feel? Though the tendency is to look at dilation and time as measures of labor's progress, these are not really measures that matter. The purpose of a contraction is to do three things: open, thin, and create descent. As long as these events are taking place, labor is progressing.

Hello, Baby!

The indication that the final hormonal shift for birthing has taken place is not so much a measure of centimeters but of behavior: you're suddenly wide awake, very focused, and in a more upright position. Now is the time to go fully into your subconscious, primal place where you can turn over everything to your body, if you're not there already.

More adrenaline enters the process to help you move your baby down and out. You may notice a change in your breathing, that it has a more high-pitched sound. You're likely to feel the urge to bear down with your contractions. Breathe through the surges for as long as you can; there's no need to push unless your body asks you to "help" at the peak of the contraction and sometimes at the tail end. You may have been feeling big pressure up to now, which is telling you that your baby is low and ready to make an entrance. Your baby is probably lower down than you might think, because you've been relaxed and you've allowed your birthing muscles to do just what they're designed to do.

Your Body Knows When to Push

The entire issue of when to push, how to push, and when to not push is confusing for birthing women and providers alike. Though the most practical approach (which also happens to be the best approach) is simply to follow what your body tells you, this also seems to be the most difficult approach to accept.

There was a time (the 1970s) when doctors believed the "hold your breath and bear down method" was the most effective and least stressful way to accommodate the baby's maneuvers to turn against the sacrum and drop beneath the pubic bone. Because fetal monitoring, new at the time, showed that the baby's heart rate dropped during these maneuvers, the belief was that the baby was in stress and had to be helped out as quickly as possible.

Research done a decade later disproved both components underpinning this approach, but beliefs and practices die hard. There are still many providers—midwives and doctors, as well as nurses in the hospital setting—who still look to the force-type pushing, and tie it to the clock or worse. And there's also the opposite, being told not to push because the doctor isn't there yet. Countless women tell of nurses yelling at them to wait to push until the doctor arrives!

The muscles that you're relying on to birth your baby are big, powerful muscles (your uterus is the biggest muscle in your body at the time of birth) and they need a lot of oxygen to do their work. Holding your breath deprives the muscle of valuable oxygen, causing lactic acid to build up and the muscles to fatigue. Bearing down when your body isn't ready for you to push is simply bearing down because there's nothing to push—nothing's ready to move. So you work for nothing. When your body signals you to push, by all means push! Now things are ready to move, and you can push with purpose. But breathe, too.

Natural Woman

Breathing techniques that help you relax also open your chest and allow your lungs to expand further. This brings more air into your lungs, and gets more oxygen into your bloodstream. The extra oxygen fuels the muscles involved in birthing—such as your uterus—so they can work at their maximum capacity. Being relaxed also helps you maintain your focus, which is crucial in the final moments of birthing.

All that maneuvering your baby does to get into the birth path does indeed stress the baby, but in positive ways. Research shows that all this twisting, turning, stretching, and compressing stimulates the baby's key systems that are complete but still in the package, so to speak. Your baby will need to use them as soon as she emerges from your body—her digestive, excretory, and respiratory systems.

Women who use hypnosis techniques and waterbirth, letting their bodies guide them, and who often breathe down, rather than push down, their babies often don't experience any change in the baby's heart rate when the baby passes under the pubic arch.

The baby is getting all the benefit of stimulation to its systems though having absolutely no oxygen-deprivation stress because both she and her mother are completely relaxed and in tune with the rhythms of their bodies and the birthing process.

Eject!

Somewhere along the birth path, there's a physiologic point that functions like an "eject" button. When your baby's head makes contact with this point, it's like flipping a switch. Suddenly your body can't get this baby out fast enough, and it's impossible for you not to push.

There's a saying that you don't have to make a river flow, it just does. It's the same thing with pushing. Your baby is going to come out … baby is not going to start kindergarten in there! A relaxed second stage is often very grunty. An observer might be thinking, "Oh, honey, you're going to have to work harder than that!" But there needs to be, and almost always is, a breath between efforts because those birthing muscles need the oxygen.

Trusty Midwife Tips

There's often a lot of yelling and carrying on when the baby starts to emerge because everyone's excited. But it's perfectly okay for you to request in your birthing preferences sheet for there to be quiet. The first sounds your baby should hear are the voices of her parents. And go for dimmed lights, too, so your baby feels that she wants to open her eyes.

Steady Does It Best

Listen to your body's tissues as you feel the baby coming out. It will feel SO BIG. This is normal. All you can do, all you should do, is let it be BIG—and breathe. It's also normal to grunt or make pushing sounds with your breathing. But it's not helpful to hold your breath, clench your teeth, and bear down like you're going to shoot your eyeballs across the room—even if you have a flash that doing so will shoot that baby right out of there and be done with it—and this will cross your mind! But it doesn't work this way. This is every bit as traumatic as it sounds; you'll do yourself some damage with this kind of pressure (like a perineal tear). And both you and your baby need the oxygen that you're withholding when you hold your breath for an extended time.

When crowning begins, imagine that you're piping your baby's name in icing onto a birthday cake during the surge of your contraction. You want a strong, steady squeeze so there are no big blobs in the middle. It's normal for you to feel that your baby's coming down, then sucking back in. Remember, there's a rhythm to contractions. This is how your body stretches your perineal tissues so they can accommodate the baby's passage without tearing. It still feels big, too big, but if you'll just let it *be* big, your body will open to accommodate it. And you'll have all those endorphins and birthing hormones to help you manage the miracle of moving a baby out of your body.

> ### Natural Woman
>
> Two-time Academy Award-winning British actor Emma Thompson conceived her daughter through in vitro fertilization, using state-of-the art technology to make pregnancy a reality for her. Then she made the commitment to a natural, nonmedicated birth. Giving birth without painkillers, she's told interviewers, is her life's greatest accomplishment. Bravo Emma!

As your baby's shoulders clear, you can reach down and take your baby. Hopefully, your baby's father is receiving and can help you bring your baby up to your chest. The baby needs to be on your chest because your chest is the best incubator and baby warmer there is; it provides just the right temperature. Having your baby on your chest also alters the receptors in your uterus, helping it to clamp down to prevent unnecessary bleeding. Anything that somebody else feels the need to do to check out the baby can be done with the baby on your chest.

Stage Three: Birthing the Placenta

Now that your baby's on your chest, safe and warm and breathing just fine, your body's ready for the final stage of labor: birthing the placenta. Your body knows the work of the placenta, which has sustained your baby all these months, is now done. The umbilical cord's been left alone to stop pulsing on its own time (more about this in Chapter 21). So contractions pick up once again, though this time not nearly as intense because they have far less of a task to accomplish. They have more of a cramplike quality, and they reach their peak within about 10 minutes. They ripple through your uterus, dislodging the placenta to begin the process of passing it from your body. It may take two or three more sessions of crampy contractions for the placenta to completely detach. This, too, is not time to be hurried along.

Sometimes providers want to hurry along this stage with a shot of Pitocin or even by tugging on the cord. If you desire, ask that your body be allowed to birth the placenta as naturally as it birthed your baby (this is something you can write in your birthing preferences). As long as there's no excessive bleeding, intervention is usually not necessary. Allowing your body to naturally birth the placenta lets the placenta peel away intact (which is what you want) and the contractions quickly allow the wall of the uterus to thicken and clamp down on itself, just as nature designed it to do.

Natural Woman

Throughout history, it's been a common practice to dry and keep the caul, or membranes, of a baby born en caul (with the amniotic membranes fully intact). The dried caul was believed to be a talisman of good fortune that would protect the child as he grew up, and would carry protective energy for all of his life. It's also a traditional practice to bury a short section of the umbilical cord at the doorway to your house, to call your child back home throughout its life.

There is good evidence for active management of the third stage of labor to prevent postpartum hemorrhage, including Pitocin after delivery of the anterior shoulder, gentle downward traction on the cord, and letting the cord pulse for 60–90 seconds before cutting. That would be the doctor's approach to avoiding a lot of bleeding. Although this is not fully in accordance with the concept of natural birth, it is still something that can be done at a homebirth if it is desired. So a person making an informed decision about what they prefer is always the best answer.

If you want to keep the placenta, most states have laws that allow you to do so. Some people want to do ceremonies that honor the placenta for having sustained a new life, such as burying it with a tree planted to celebrate the baby's birth. In some cultures, the placenta has medicinal uses. Some people consume a portion of the placenta as a means of heading off postpartum depression, increasing milk supply, and helping the body to heal more quickly. And if you don't want to keep the placenta, that's fine, too—most women are content to let the midwife, birthing center, or hospital appropriately dispose of it.

Oh, Baby!

If you're intending to consume the placenta, it is important to handle it carefully and to chill or freeze it as quickly as possible. Your doula is a good person to put in charge of this responsibility. She can place the placenta in a food freezer bag and put it into a cooler with ice, or straight into the freezer if a homebirth. Examination of the placenta is standard procedure in hospitals and many birthing centers, so let your practitioner know in advance of the birth that you intend to keep the placenta. Placental consumption is not a good idea if you have hepatitis, HIV/AIDS, or other bloodborne or infectious diseases.

The Bigness of Birth

Birth is big. It's the biggest thing you'll ever do, and it's the biggest thing you'll ever feel in your body, and leaving your body. Yet nobody teaches us how to honor the bigness of birth. Instead, it's our cultural perspective to make birth smaller, so it looks and feels more like something we can handle. Every woman faces that moment of truth when she sees beyond this curtain, sees the big, and thinks, "How is that ever going to get out of me?" Choosing a nonmedicated birth requires a leap of faith that puts your trust in the design of your body and its ability to handle the bigness of birthing.

Natural, nonmedicated birth can happen in about 85 to 90 percent of births. We know this not through speculation, conjecture, or extrapolations of wishful thinking but through worldwide documented experience in countries such as Denmark where natural, nonmedicated birth is the norm. When the natural processes of birth are allowed to unfold, only about 10 to 15 percent of births require medical attention or intervention. Yet we culturally equate something that can hurt with something being wrong. In birth, this is the wrong equation; in birth, this is simply not true. However, it is the belief we hold, collectively, about birth, and all efforts to prepare for birth emphasize reducing the pain.

When you feel comfortable, there just isn't as much pain in your body; many women who choose nonmedicated birth say that though they do feel intense pressure, they don't perceive it as pain. Comfort has many layers, however, and is often about more than the relaxation, hypnosis, water, and other methods you use. Sometimes discomfort arises from being in unfamiliar surroundings. It might take time to settle in to feel safe and at ease. Continuous interruptions, however well intended, may so challenge your ability to settle in that you can't or never do. The tension you feel fills your body, and before long it becomes impossible to relax and center yourself.

Birth is instinctive and primitive; for many women, the connection with this primal part of themselves surfaces somewhere around 9 centimeters. This is well beyond the point of options, and it can be scary to think we might put ourselves out there, counting on this connection to pull us through, and then somehow miss making it. Think, though, of the joy you'll feel when you can make the connection!

The only time in life that we get agitated is when we can't let go of how we think things should be and instead look at how things are. We hang on to expectations, even when doing so doesn't serve us very well and even when we know better. Your positive visualizations are important, but you also must remain in the current moment. Sometimes you do need to cry or go in the shower and yell, so you can let go. Partners want to say, "hang on, honey," but sometimes they should say, "let go, baby." When you let go of old ideas and expectations, you're free to make the connection with your primal self and your natural birth is free to unfold on its own agenda.

The Least You Need to Know

♦ Use what you know when you want to use it; it's counterproductive to save your most effective methods for later.

♦ Your body has built-in mechanisms to move your baby out.

♦ The timing of birth has nothing to do with the time on the clock.

♦ Letting go will take you closer to your best birth than will holding on.

Chapter 20

What if the Pain Is Too Much ... and Other Things That Can Happen

In This Chapter

- ◆ When nothing you try works
- ◆ Medication options: pain relievers and the epidural
- ◆ No more progress
- ◆ Having your best birth when a c-section becomes necessary

Birth has its own agenda. And when that agenda dovetails with your hopes and expectations, it's hard to remember this. So when birth takes off on its own trajectory, it often catches you by surprise. All that talk about a backup plan—well, that was for everyone else in the childbirth class, not you! But things happen sometimes that no one can predict or control.

If your birth takes off on its own orbit, stay calm and stay flexible. You have backup preparations for a reason, and that's just as important as anything else you've done to be ready for your birth. You're still only a short time away from holding your beautiful baby joyfully in your arms. And you don't necessarily have to give up your intention to have a natural birth. You only have to stay flexible and open-minded … and sometimes a little bit creative.

More Than You Bargained For

Severe pain during birthing is a red flag that maybe something's not right. When all the methods you've learned cannot provide relaxation and comfort, it's time for a closer look to see what's going on. Birth is intense, yes. But no woman should ever be in *intense* pain. Part of trusting yourself involves knowing that what you're experiencing has moved beyond what's normal. Sometimes when you're feeling a lot of pain, especially in early labor, it's because you're tense. Maybe you're distracted by other people or by your surroundings such that you can't find your focus. You may also be holding doubts about whether you can really trust your body and this process of birth. Fear makes it very difficult to relax. When you can't relax, you end up fighting your contractions—and that hurts. This is the fear-tension-pain cycle we talked about in Chapter 4, and over time it becomes self-perpetuating.

It's a natural response to become despairing of being able to pull yourself back once you hit that point where all you can think about is how much the next contraction is going to hurt. If you find yourself struggling to relax, before you ask for pain relief medications or an epidural, give the water one more try. A birthing tub is best because you can submerge nearly your entire body. A regular bathtub filled to the max can sometimes be an acceptable substitute if you can get the water level to the middle of your belly.

If you don't have a tub of any kind, get in the shower. The shower works wonders— it's small, so you feel cocooned and protected. The sound of the running water is relaxing and hypnotic, and the warm water on your body feels good, minimizes the feelings of pain, and increases your relaxation. The water hitting your nipples can make your labor more effective, and thus shorter, by stimulating your body to release more oxytocin. Put a towel on the birthing ball, sit down in the shower, and feel free to camp out in there!

No matter what your fears and worries, being in the water in this way removes 75 percent of the effect of gravity. That's not just in your head, either; it's a law of physics. You can't help but relax when three fourths of the pressure against your body goes away. If, after 20 minutes or so in the water, you still feel a lot of pain, ask your provider to do a thorough examination to determine whether things are as they should be—not just the routine vaginal exam to check your cervix, but a good going-over to evaluate possible reasons for why you feel the way you do.

It's important to trust that your body may be telling you something's not quite right. A common situation is that the baby's head isn't lined up properly. Your provider or a good doula can suggest position changes that are specific to the baby's location to help move him into a better position for birthing. Your labor will then feel better, and the baby can "get on with it."

Trusty Midwife Tips

When you feel yourself at the edge of your tolerance, consider asking for the lights to be dimmed (if they're not already) and for 30 minutes of no interruptions or conversation. Your doula might sit outside your door to remind others that this is your "time out." Having a lot of people bustling around is distracting under the best of circumstances. Asking them to step out or stay quiet can give you the space you need to calm yourself and refocus your energy. And this can allow your labor to progress very well.

A Crunch Start

One of the most common reasons for pain in early labor is a baby who's in an awkward position. Sometimes the baby's position will self-correct as labor progresses. Depending on how far the baby has dropped and where you are in your labor, a skilled midwife or doctor can manually maneuver the baby into a more amenable position. You will have to marshal all your relaxation skills to let your body be helped by someone else's fingers. And sometimes you're going to need more help to birth the baby. Your doctor may recommend an epidural to give your body a break so you can relax enough for the baby to reposition.

Occasionally, an especially intense early labor means you're having an unusually fast labor. Your provider's examination will reveal this if it's the case, because your cervix will be far more open than would be typical in early labor. Knowing that this is what is happening is often enough to give you the resolve to continue your natural methods (especially hypnotic techniques and the birthing tub), because although your contractions are hurting, you can just relax one thing more in your body and know you'll be done soon. You have a very efficient set of birthing muscles—lucky you!

Too Much, Too Long

Active labor requires intense focus and energy from you, and a long active phase can be very tiring. This is why you need to continue eating and drinking throughout your labor. Pain relief medications become very enticing when you're exhausted. You may indeed be at the end of your ability to cope; an injection of a narcotic pain relief medication could give you the rest you need to recover so you can return to labor with renewed strength and focus.

The narcotic fentanyl is often favored at the end of labor because it's fast-acting, highly effective, and then gone quickly from your body so it won't be in the baby's system, either. However, doctors do usually save fentanyl for the end because your body responds less with each administration of it. Morphine is also very effective for pain relief, but it is a muscle relaxant and does slow labor. Many women fall right asleep with morphine and then forget that they're in labor or even at a hospital. Each contraction comes as a fresh surprise, which can make you feel very out of control.

Oh, Baby!

If you're intending to birth at a birthing center, make sure you know the center's policies for medications. Some medical model birthing centers may offer pain relief medications and Pitocin; others do not. Midwifery model birthing centers do not provide medications, although they're especially experienced in using nonmedical methods to help birthing women achieve relaxation and comfort. With homebirth, pain medications are not an option; drugs of any kind are medical interventions that alter the body's natural processes and necessitate medical supervision.

The Medication Decision

When you've planned and prepared for a natural, nonmedicated birth, it's often difficult to make the choice to accept pain relief medications. If you've tried your best and you've made all the decisions yourself along the way about what to try next, then you know you've truly reached this intersection without letting someone else hijack your birth. You've done all you can, and that's all you can do. Pain relief medications are simply other options to consider now so you can continue with your intent to have the best birth possible.

When you decide you want medications for pain relief, you do step with both feet into the medical model. This means that if you've chosen homebirth and you decide you want pain medications, your midwife will arrange for you to be transported to a birthing center or hospital; this should be part of your birthing preferences and something you've agreed upon in advance.

Many doctors and hospitals have an open approach toward pain relief medications and are willing to help you work your way back to a natural birth; some are not, and crossing the medication line becomes a point of no return with regard to the level of control or even participation you can have in the remainder of your birthing. The medications themselves often establish the scenario of a medical birth because they alter the flow and rhythm of labor. Your body may simply abdicate to them. Labor slows or stops, and further interventions become necessary to bring the birth to completion. And all this help does mean that now both you and the baby must be monitored, all the time, until birth.

 Oh, Baby!

When it's late in labor and you're considering pain relief medication, ask to be checked *before* taking the medication so you know how dilated you are. If you're at 8 or 9 centimeters, birth is imminent and you may choose to stay with your natural relaxation methods for this final stretch.

An important factor to consider when you're deciding about medications for pain relief is that they're tied to certain markers in the progression of your labor. Generally speaking, you can't have an epidural before 4 centimeters and you can't have narcotic medications after 8 centimeters. Except for an epidural, there are also time considerations for how frequently you can receive pain relief medications—every two to three hours is the common frequency.

Knowing these parameters may help restore your confidence in your body and your ability to continue with a nonmedicated birth, particularly if you've reached the 8-centimeter mark and you know you're within an hour or two of birthing your baby. Sometimes this knowledge is enough to renew your focus, and you can use your natural methods for the short time—relatively speaking—that remains in your labor. Your own situation is unique, of course, and you'll need to work closely with your doctor to make decisions about medications that are specific and appropriate for you.

Narcotic Medications

Narcotic pain relief medications work by attaching to the same receptors that endorphins use. Narcotics have a stronger binding ability than endorphins and can flood the receptors very rapidly because the drug enters your system in a bolus (or mass). The effect both blocks the transmission of pain signals from nerves to your brain and makes you sleepy—very sleepy. By this time, sleep is good—so a nap is often highly restorative. The narcotic pain relief medications most commonly used in labor are morphine and fentanyl, usually administered by IV injection. Their effectiveness typically lasts one to three hours.

Narcotic drugs are also powerful muscle relaxants. This is helpful when you've become exhausted, which is usually the case, because the chemical relaxation inherently releases some of the tension in your body. The downside is that the relaxation effect slows contractions—and your uterus, too, is a big muscle. And it might really appreciate the opportunity to stop working for a while.

Your uterus can return to labor when the narcotic's effect wears off, rested and recharged. Sometimes your uterus can't or doesn't, though—it's lost its rhythm and momentum. Then your doctor may suggest Pitocin (synthetic oxytocin) to boost your labor back up and keep it going. Pitocin-stimulated contractions tend to be sharp and intense, lacking in the smooth rhythm that characterizes natural contractions. So with Pitocin, you often need additional or continued pain relief medications. An often unanticipated "side effect" of narcotic drugs is that they can start an intervention cascade. Knowing this can happen is your best defense for heading it off by carefully evaluating all suggested interventions so you can make fully informed decisions about them.

Some women can have a Pitocin-driven labor without any pain relief drugs. These women have good support, possibly more than one person there to help through every contraction. It can be done, but you are the only one who can decide what is right for you and your baby. Narcotic drugs, like most substances that enter your body, do cross the placenta—so they also affect your baby. They can slow the baby's heart rate during labor and can depress the baby's respiratory reflex at birth if the drug is still in the baby's system.

The Epidural

An epidural is a form of regional anesthesia, and only an anesthesiologist (a physician specialist) can administer it. You must be in a hospital to have an epidural. The anesthesiologist inserts a needle with a tiny catheter into the space around your spinal cord in the small of your back, the needle is removed, and the tiny, flexible, tubelike catheter stays to deliver a numbing drug and often a narcotic pain reliever. An epidural blocks pain signals from traveling up your spinal cord to your brain.

A conventional epidural also blocks the nerves that move your legs, so there's no getting out of bed once the epidural is in place. The catheter stays in place until after your baby is born (you won't feel it or even be aware that it's there). A modified form of epidural, commonly called a "walking epidural," uses less medication so you can still have control of your leg muscles. However, you're not all that likely to do much walking because you have an IV and probably continuous fetal monitoring. The drugs used in epidurals can have a range of effects on you and on your baby, so doctors will closely monitor both of you once the epidural has been administered.

> **Oh, Baby!** _____
>
> Do you have a tattoo on your lower back? Some anesthesiologists will not perform an epidural if they have to insert the needle through the tattoo. Although the generally accepted standard is that a tattoo is fully healed in six months, there are anesthesiologists who feel there is still a risk for tiny fragments of ink to break away when the needle penetrates the tattoo and be carried into the space around the spinal cord. If you have a lower-back tattoo, discuss with your doctor whether it will affect your ability to have an epidural.

There's the perception that an epidural takes away all the sensations of labor. This isn't quite true. An epidural blocks pain signals from making it to your brain. But the contractions continue, and you still feel the intensity of their pressure. In some ways, this experience is not much different than the effect of deep hypnosis combined with the birthing tub. You feel the pressure, but there is no pain. Even with an epidural, you can and should continue to use the methods of relaxation and focus that you learned to prepare for your birth. This is still your birth, and your thoughts, emotions, and actions continue to shape how it unfolds.

Although relatively safe overall, the epidural nonetheless has the potential for side effects and complications—some of which can be serious. Many women experience a drop in blood pressure 20 to 30 minutes after the epidural starts, which causes the baby's heart rate to drop. The baby usually recovers, although the nurses may ask you to roll on one side and then the other and may also put an oxygen mask on your face and have you breathe deeply to increase the level of oxygen in your blood. Occasionally, the baby cannot recover quickly enough, and a c-section right away becomes the best option.

> **Oh, Baby!** _____
>
> Although an epidural is a relatively safe intervention, it's important to remember that it is an invasive procedure with some significant potential risks, including excessive bleeding and permanent spinal cord damage. And it is anesthesia; only an anesthesiologist (a physician with specialized training and credentials) can perform an epidural. Many health experts are concerned that women are not receiving full information about the risks of epidural and therefore are not able to make appropriately knowledgeable decisions.

One of the most confounding, delayed side effects of an epidural is that women who have epidurals tend to develop fevers postpartum. This presents a dilemma for the doctor, because there's also the specter of an infection. So you'll find yourself the subject of much poking, prodding, and testing to determine whether there is a medical condition underlying your fever. Many doctors simply prescribe a course of antibiotics to cover all the bases. Your baby, too, will also be subject to close scrutiny and likely a "work up" to make sure all is well. Make sure you fully understand what this involves and the reasons for doing it.

> **Trusty Midwife Tips**
>
> An epidural may provide instant and dramatic relief, but the price tag for the relatively short duration of its use may give you sticker shock. According to a 2009 article in *The Wall Street Journal*, the total bill for an epidural is close to $4,000—for equipment and supplies, the drugs, and the anesthesiologist's services. Even if you have health insurance that picks up 70 to 80 percent of the cost, you could be looking at an $800 bill—about $300 or $400 per hour for pain relief. Not that you should decline an epidural on the basis of its cost, but it is a factor to consider when you're considering your options.

Another challenging side effect comes during postpartum—your milk coming in. Having an epidural delays milk production by about the same length of time as you have the epidural. If you have an eight- or twelve-hour epidural, your milk will come in at the end of the third day postpartum rather than at the start. You'll still produce colostrum (the energy-rich "premilk") during this time, although your baby will be ready for your milk on nature's schedule.

The medications used for an epidural also cross the placenta and affect the baby, although not to the same extent as narcotic pain medications injected into the mother's bloodstream. The drugs may remain in the baby's system for up to seven days because his liver isn't quite up to the task of breaking them down so his body can process and eliminate them as waste.

Laboring Down with an Epidural

When you have an epidural during the birthing phase of labor, you're likely to need the guidance of your partner and midwife or doctor to coordinate your conscious efforts (such as pushing) with your contractions. The chemical relaxation of the epidural means that you're not aware of the urge to push; the nerves that would bring that urge to your attention are blocked from carrying impulses. This makes it more likely that your body will need help from you, in the form of intentional pushing, to help move the baby along in its descent. Often, you'll be told when you are having a contraction—and you'll get lots of verbal help in how to make the most of it.

Because an epidural interrupts the natural flow of labor, it alters the hormonal cocktail. You may not have as potent a blend of hormones as you otherwise would, meaning you have to draw more from your conscious mind to coordinate with your body's efforts. Breathing your baby down, as you would do with hypnotic techniques and the birthing tub, is still possible but requires strong concentration on your part—along with lots of encouragement from your birth support team. Once the baby begins crowning or is at the perineum, you'll have to do some pushing to get your baby birthed.

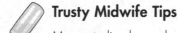

Trusty Midwife Tips

Many studies have shown it really works to labor down. Waiting for maybe one to two hours, even, after a woman is fully dilated—until the baby's head can be seen at the vaginal opening or until the woman feels a sensation like she needs to bear down even with the epidural—can help reduce the amount of time pushing.

Failure to Progress

The most common reason for intervention in birthing is broadly termed "failure to progress." This can mean such a range of circumstances that the term really has little substance. Its effect, however, is to tie your labor—and specifically your cervical dilation—to the clock. Your midwife or doctor may tell you that if your dilation does not increase in two hours, it will then be necessary to intervene.

If you find yourself in such a situation, do your best to relax. Use your meditation and visualization methods to "see" your contractions opening your cervix and to help your body find its best opportunity for resuming a natural birth. Sometimes "failure to progress" is more about failure to be patient and failure to wait for nature to take its course; especially if you've received any medication, your labor is on the clock. Sometimes, however, failure to progress is just that, and you will know—or sense—that it is time to accept whatever interventions are necessary for your baby's best birth.

My, What a Big Baby You Have

Cephalopelvic disproportion, or CPD, is a commonly cited reason for surgical birth. This means that the baby's head cannot maneuver through the mother's pelvis, usually presented as "the baby's head is too big." A large baby isn't necessarily more difficult to birth; as earlier chapters discuss, a larger baby is often easier to birth because its mass more quickly and surely activates the mechanisms along the birth path that propel it along.

As well, the pelvis has an amazing capacity to flex and open. All through your pregnancy, your hormones have been at work to soften ligaments just for this reason. Your pelvis has four bones that meet with tissue designed to stretch. Your pelvis will become huge. Your baby's head has five bones that are designed to overlap during the pressures of birth, so the head will become smaller … it's all designed to work just fine.

Some women do have unusually narrow or small pelvic openings, though, and there may be a disproportion between the ability of the pelvis to open and the size of the baby. A woman may also have structural anomalies that alter the way her pelvic bones align with one another. When such circumstances exist, a c-section is usually the only option. However, it will take until the pushing phase of labor before anyone can honestly determine whether this is true. Telling you at four centimeters that you have CPD is just not possible.

Bottom's Down

Hey, that's not a head! Sometimes your baby has a surprise for you: breech position. Most of the time, your midwife or doctor can feel that the baby is in a head-up position near the time of birth. A fair number of babies are in a breech position until two weeks or so before birth, then they turn and settle into the head-down position. Some babies wait until labor is well underway before deciding to turn head down, though.

Some doctors consider a breech birth to be an automatic c-section. The baby's head is what normally opens the way for the rest of the body, especially the shoulders. Doctors worry that a breech birth may result in the baby getting stuck, necessitating an emergency c-section. So they prefer to sidestep the issue by scheduling the birth as a c-section or converting it to such when the breech is discovered.

Sometimes getting onto your hands and knees nudges the baby to turn itself head-down. Using a slant-board with your head down (or trying Hatha yoga's Downward-Facing Dog pose), acupuncture, homeopathics, and hypnosis also have a good track record for helping your baby turn before birth day. Some midwives and doctors are able to manipulate the baby into turning, although manipulated babies have the propensity to turn themselves right back. This is called aversion and is most successfully done at about 37 weeks. A breech presentation should not inherently rule out a natural birth, although how far you get with this depends on the skill and comfort level of your practitioner.

When your baby is in a breech presentation, it is essential not to push until half the baby's body is birthed. This takes enormous concentration. Then, once half the body is out, you have to push, push, and push until the head pops out. Some babies born breech need a few minutes of rescue breathing to get the urge to breathe on their own, although again this is something the staff are trained and prepared to do.

Oops, I Pooped

Little silences a roomful of chatty hospital or birthing center staff like the appearance of meconium staining—streaks of the goopy, greenish, tarlike substance coating the inside of your baby's intestines until birth that float out with the amniotic fluid after the amniotic membranes rupture. Most babies have their first bowel movements, during which they pass the meconium, in the first days following birth. About one in five doesn't wait—passing meconium before birth.

Meconium discharge can be a sign that the baby is experiencing distress (nonreassuring fetal status or nonreassuring heart tones, hospital staff will say)—not getting enough oxygen. However, most babies born with meconium staining are not in distress and have no ill effects. No one really knows why some babies release meconium before birth, and there isn't any sure way to know whether meconium discharge means a distressed baby.

Light meconium staining is usually no big deal—only a bit messy. Heavy meconium staining is potentially more serious. The risk is that the baby may inhale some meconium into his lungs, setting up what's called meconium aspiration syndrome. The meconium, because it's so thick and sticky, can block the baby's airways and is very difficult to remove. It's this risk that turns the mood when meconium appears, and the more meconium the higher the risk. A baby that inhales meconium may need treatment ranging from suctioning the meconium out right at birth to antibiotics and occasionally mechanical ventilation (a breathing machine) until his lungs can properly inflate and function.

When It Comes to C-Section

In about 10 to 12 percent of births, according to the World Health Organization's standards, a c-section is a necessary intervention. Should you turn out to be among this 10 to 12 percent, there are still ways you can remain an active and aware participant in the birth. An epidural is the usual form of anesthesia for c-section; it allows you to be awake and carries less risk for both you and your baby. You won't feel any pain from the surgery, although you will feel pressure and tugging.

Trusty Midwife Tips _____

It's typical procedure during a c-section to put a fabric screen between your head and the rest of your body. You may assume this is to keep you from seeing what's going on, but the primary reason is that the screen establishes the sterile field where the surgery is taking place. In reality, you can't see what's happening at your belly when you're lying flat on your back, anyway!

Nearly always your partner can be present during the c-section. Ask the obstetrician to let you touch, or at least see, your baby as she's born. Most will do this as long as there are no medical issues with the baby. If there are, and the staff are intending to whisk the baby away to address those medical concerns, ask for your partner to be able to go with the baby. (These are things you can, and should, cover in your birthing preferences; see Chapter 17.)

With an uneventful c-section, you should be able to have your baby as soon as you are in recovery. With help, you can nurse your baby at this time. Your baby will be with you as you are moved from recovery to your postpartum room. Unless your baby has medical concerns, you should be able to have your baby in your room with you until you go home.

Oh, Baby! _____

One in eight babies is born before 37 weeks in the United States, nearly half of them due to induced labor or c-section. A study reported in 2009 revealed the surprising and alarming finding that these babies have a much higher rate of learning difficulties than babies born full-term. The finding suggests that much more brain growth and development of the brain takes place in the final weeks of pregnancy than doctors realized, and has resulted in a collective recommendation to end elective inductions and c-sections before 39 weeks.

Take a "Pass" on the Guilt Trip

When you've worked hard to shape your birth experience but it goes a different direction, it's easy to feel disappointed and wonder whether you could have done just one more thing for everything to get back on track. Could you have done things differently? Maybe. Would it have made a difference in the way things unfolded? Highly unlikely. We go back to where we started in this chapter: birth has its own agenda. You've worked hard, and you've given your best for yourself and for your baby. Your baby knows this, your partner knows this, and your midwife knows this. Everybody knows this! So let yourself know it, too.

The Least You Need to Know

◆ Medications and interventions are options to consider to help you have your best birth when things are not going as you expected.

◆ A single injection of a narcotic pain relief medication is often enough to let your body relax and rest so you can then resume your natural birth.

◆ Sometimes an epidural affects the baby's heart rate, making an immediate c-section necessary.

◆ When you participate in all the decisions that affect the course of your birth, you're doing everything possible to make your best birth happen.

Part 6

Welcoming Your New Baby

When you're calm and relaxed during birth, your baby is, too. Forget the stereotypical wailing scream! Your baby's awake, alert, and curious to meet you. Your baby wants to go right from your womb to your arms … and that's how it should be (no whisking away to be weighed and measured). And what would you think if we told you now, as kind of a sneak peek, that you are very likely to be up and around and feeling pretty much like yourself even within hours of birthing? You won't believe what a difference it makes when you work *with* your body's natural rhythms and efforts to let the birth unfold on its own agenda! These final chapters talk about the culminating experience of a natural birth and what you might expect during the first few weeks afterward—for you, for your baby, and for your partner and other family members as you all settle into your new roles.

21

Your Baby's First Moments, Naturally

In This Chapter

- ◆ What babies remember of their births
- ◆ Skin-to-skin contact between mother and baby soon after birth is important for bonding
- ◆ The changes your baby undergoes in the first hours following birth
- ◆ Endorphins for you and for your baby

The first moments after birth are sacred. You and your baby are meeting, skin to skin and eye to eye, for the first time. Although the tendency of those in attendance is to rush to make sure the baby is okay, what's more important is to savor the miracle of new life. In his first minute out of your womb, your baby should hear only the voices of his parents, feel only the touch of his parents, and smell only the scents of his parents.

The lights should be dim so he will open his eyes and look at you. The room should be still and warm so he feels calm and safe. This time is so precious; although it passes in what seems like a heartbeat, it will live in your heart and soul in such a way that when you close your eyes, you're there again. And the same goes for your baby, who will remember those first moments as ones of loving welcome. You and your partner will speak to your child of these first moments after birth with reverence, joy, and love for the rest of your life. Your baby will turn to you to put into words the memories he cannot express: the story of his birth.

What an Amazing Thing You've Done!

Look what you've done! Isn't it so amazing? Your baby rests peacefully on your chest, taking in all she has experienced in recent hours. She's alert, aware, and awake. So are you. Whatever doubts or tiredness you were feeling even minutes ago has evaporated, and such a glowing euphoria emanates from you that everyone in the room feels it, too, and smiles. It doesn't seem quite possible, yet here you are—holding your baby in your arms. And nothing should come between the two of you until you feel ready to move. There's no need to rush to weigh and measure the baby; she's not going to grow in the next few hours. It's more important that the two of you get to know each other and establish the bonding that's so essential for both of you.

Trusty Midwife Tips

Bringing your baby to your chest immediately after he's born helps to reassure him that everything is still familiar and safe. Your chest is warm, and your baby can hear and feel your heartbeat and breathing. These are calming, comforting experiences. And you feel your baby's heartbeat and breathing, too, which is greatly reassuring.

Onto Your Chest

The skin-to-skin contact of your baby lying on your chest is important for both of you. You should receive your baby immediately onto your chest when he is born; the umbilical cord is usually plenty long enough to reach, and if it's a little short, on your belly is good, too. Women who have had a natural, nonmedicated birth—especially a homebirth or a waterbirth—are sometimes so internally focused that they appear disoriented and confused at the time of birth and in the moments right after.

Your partner or midwife can gently tell you to reach down and take your baby and pull him to your chest. Australian natural birth guru and physician Sarah Buckley (author of the natural birth classic *Gentle Birth, Gentle Mothering*, now in its third edition) refers to this as the woman has checked out of her body and is up in the stars retrieving the soul of her baby. To the outside observer, this is pretty much how it looks!

Sometimes in a hospital birth, the midwife or doctor keeps the baby down between the mom's legs to clean and suction the baby. Often, this is only because it's the routine of how the hospital does things, although sometimes it has to do with the practitioner's beliefs about cord clamping (more about this a few pages later in this chapter). If you've arranged for your partner to receive the baby, then you've bypassed the entire issue before anyone can object. If your partner is not receiving the baby, either or both of you can speak up at the moment of birth to get the baby onto mom's chest.

Your chest is a natural incubator, adjusting your baby's temperature when it changes by even a quarter of a degree to keep him at precisely the right degree of warmth. When your baby is lying on your chest, it just so happens that his head is right under your nose. This is part of birth's design. The smell of your baby stimulates your body to change, one more time, its hormonal mix. This triggers more receptors in the uterus, causing it to clamp down and birth the placenta usually less than an hour following the baby's birth.

> **Trusty Midwife Tips**
>
> If you need or want a blanket following your baby's birth, have someone put it over you and your baby together, preserving your skin-to-skin contact. This signals your baby that she's still safe; she's not being separated from you. And as long as your baby's lying on your chest, she doesn't need one of those little hats or any clothes to keep her warm. It's more important that the two of you have enough "skin time" to complete the bonding process.

First Breath

A baby's first breath is four times the tidal volume (pressure in the lungs) than any other breath the baby will ever take. Some babies don't take a first breath right away, however, which often generates a sense of controlled panic in the room. As long as the umbilical cord remains attached to the baby and pulsing, though, the baby's getting blood and therefore oxygen—just like he has for his entire life. And nearly all babies will start to breathe on their own within a minute of birth.

Heart rate is the key to the baby's status; as long as it remains strong and high enough, the baby is fine and will take a breath when she's ready. Some babies have a lot of amniotic fluid in their lungs when they're born, which makes that first breath a little harder to take. Occasionally, a baby does need help with its first breath. This may mean a minute or two of rescue breathing, and then the baby breathes on her own.

Oh, Baby! _____

Although rescue breathing sounds a little scary, it's really just a way to give your new infant's breathing a nudge. Sometimes the midwife or doctor may administer a small amount of oxygen, too, to give a boost to the oxygen level of the baby's blood.

Unclamped and Uncut

Ideally, the cord remains unclamped and uncut until it stops pulsing—typically about five minutes. This allows the blood in the cord to finish redistributing from the placenta and cord to the baby. When the cord stops pulsing, your baby is breathing on his own, has a stable blood volume, and no longer needs the oxygen coming to him through the umbilical cord. So your body then naturally begins the final contractions to separate and birth the placenta. This is called a physiologic third stage—there is no medical intervention to initiate or assist with the placenta's expulsion. In a physiologic third stage, the cord often is not clamped and cut until after the placenta is birthed.

There is controversy about delayed cord clamping. It has become the standard practice of medical birth in the United States to clamp the cord within seconds of the baby emerging from the birth path. This stems from the view that the baby needs to remain below the level of the mother's heart after birth to prevent too much blood from flowing into its body—a situation called hypertransfusion, which can lead to a disorder called polycythemia.

Oh, Baby! _____

About one in eight babies born in the United States develops polycythemia; there are numerous possible causes, and often no clear cause is identified. The health risk of polycythemia is that the overabundance of red blood cells makes the blood too thick (hyperviscous), and it cannot properly flow through the lungs. Treatment approaches for polycythemia in newborns are controversial, with studies showing that they may not affect the outcome. Fortunately, most babies who develop polycythemia recover. Babies who are polycythemic can also have more problems with jaundice as newborns.

Though a number of studies challenge this belief, it remains a tenet of medical birth in the United States. In a hospital setting, a doctor or midwife may agree to a delay of 60 to 90 seconds, but not often any longer. However, delayed cord clamping is the standard in numerous other countries including Australia and Denmark.

The placenta and the umbilical cord are structures that belong to the baby and contain only the baby's blood. As much as one third of the baby's blood supply is in the placenta and cord at the time of birth. Whether in favor of or opposed to delayed cord clamping, both sides observe that allowing even four to five minutes before clamping the cord lets more of the blood redistribute to the baby's body, increasing the baby's supply of oxygen-bearing red blood cells as well as approximately two tablespoons of stem cells.

You Smell So Good!

The smell of your baby is important to stimulate your body to change its hormonal mix so you can wrap up this birth. The vernix caseosa that coats your baby's body—a waxy, dense slathering of oils and sloughed cells from your baby's skin—is loaded with pheromones, odorless chemicals that your primal self reacts to as though you could smell them. The vernix also has a distinct, although faint, odor. In the womb, the vernix protected your baby's skin from the amniotic fluid in which he floated, so it carries the smells of your baby's total existence.

Birth attendants are often quick to attempt to "clean up" the baby, but there is no reason to do this right away. There's nothing harmful or damaging about vernix; your baby has been wearing this protective coating for a long time. It will massage into the baby's skin with movement and handling. There's no real need for a bath just yet.

You also give off pheromones and odors that trigger bonding instincts in your baby. The effect of this is strongest during the 12 hours immediately following birth. You may feel like you want to clean yourself up, even take a shower, after the birth. But to preserve your smell, you should wait—or at least shower only from the waist down. All the smells that may be concerning you, like your armpits, are vital to the bonding that's taking place. The smell of your breasts, too, is particularly important for your baby. It's worthwhile to wait to wash yourself and your baby. Your midwife or doula can help you take a sponge bath after an hour or two.

The Sea Change of Your Baby's First 12 Hours

If we adults had to do what a newborn has to do in the first five minutes following birth, we couldn't do it. It's an enormous shift to leave the womb and enter the world. Everything about how the baby looks, feels, and behaves changes. It's more work for your baby to be "on land"; remember our mantra about water relieving 75 percent of gravity's pressure? Well, your baby has been floating in water all his life!

Coming into the pressurized world means his body must now work harder. His body is ready for the transition, of course; the process of birthing helps lay in the final preparations. But we can't help but believe it has to be quite a challenge for him to wrap his thoughts around this new world he's suddenly in as he's adapting to his new environment.

Natural Woman

Did you know that all newborns look like their fathers at birth? This is so the father knows the baby is his and is willing to care for and protect it; the mother already knows it's hers because she's carried the baby inside her. Most babies change appearance dramatically over the first three days following birth, establishing their own "look."

The Body Dynamic

Physically, your baby is using for the first time most of her major body systems; she had no need for them in the womb when your body systems did all the work. But now she breathes, eats, poops, and pees—her respiratory, digestive, excretory, and elimination systems are now working on their own. Even her cardiovascular and nervous systems, which did function before birth, have changed significantly to accommodate life in the outside world.

Your baby opens her eyes although she can focus on objects only within an eight- to twelve-inch range from her face. Her senses of smell and taste are still very basic, except for her ability to detect noxious smells and bitter tastes. These are defensive mechanisms that cause her to automatically attempt to get away from potentially harmful substances; these are reflexes she'll have all her life, although she'll learn other ways to identify things that are not good for her, such as spoiled food and poisonous substances. She's pretty wide awake for her first 12 to 24 hours out of the womb, taking in as much of this new environment as she can absorb. She'll sleep, then, on and off for most of the next 24 hours, so you may need to wake her for feedings. (Although some babies are the opposite and are sleepy in the first 24 hours and wide awake in the second.)

Your baby should be at your breast within 20 minutes of birth, although probably it'll seem like she's more playing around than putting any effort into breastfeeding (Chapter 23 is all about breastfeeding). This is not only normal and good; it's essential. Babies have an inborn instinct to root and suck. Even making contact with your nipple, however brief, affirms this instinct and strengthens her efforts. Nonmedicated babies will latch at 20 to 30 minutes after birth if the breast is near. Some will latch sooner, and some may need that first hour to "get" it—but all will latch unless something else is going on.

Trusty Midwife Tips _____

There's a common perception that newborns can't see very well. This isn't quite true. Newborns are very nearsighted for the first two weeks, able to focus on things within about 15 inches. But within that distance, a baby can focus sharply. It's no accident that this is just about the distance between your face and your baby's face when you're breastfeeding! Babies are drawn to faces, and will focus on them when they come in range. Adults might instinctively cue into this when they bend down to coo at the baby!

Some hospitals have a standard practice of giving a newborn a little bit of "sugar water" (glucose solution) to provide a boost of energy, on the premise that the baby uses a lot of energy during birth. However, she's been receiving full nourishment through the umbilical cord right up until the time the cord stops pulsing or is clamped and cut.

The giving of glucose is something to discuss with the baby's doctor; ask whether the baby has any indications of low blood sugar or dehydration. Though these circumstances can occur, they're not true of every baby. Glucose supplementation may not be necessary and can lessen your baby's interest in breastfeeding. It also means processed sugar is what goes first into your baby's intestines.

If your baby is showing good interest in your breasts, that's where you want her attention focused for receiving nourishment and hydration. Your colostrum, the thick fluid in your breasts for the first three days after birthing, is highly concentrated—so very small amounts deliver high nutritional value. This is all that most babies need. It's like baby yogurt!

Testing, Testing

When your birth takes place in a hospital or birthing center, your baby typically undergoes a battery of tests and procedures in the first 24 to 96 hours following birth. First, of course, is the weighing and measuring. Although these are considered vital statistics for helping to assess your baby's health, they're not going to change if you wait a few hours.

Most states mandate babies to be tested for low thyroid (because hypothyroidism at birth can cause serious, irreversible mental and physical impairments) and the metabolic disorder phenylketonuria (PKU), which also has lifelong implications. These tests, although valuable, can wait until you are ready to leave the hospital or birth center; they don't need to be done in the first hours of life. If you've chosen homebirth, your midwife usually can collect the blood samples or you can have them done through the baby's health-care provider.

States may also mandate testing for other metabolic disorders, because many are treatable with early detection. Such mandatory testing is controversial, however. Many states also require newborns to receive injections of vitamin K, a clotting factor, and hepatitis vaccine as well as antibiotic ointment in the eyes.

> **Oh, Baby!** _____
>
> If you choose to decline routine measures such as eye antibiotic and vitamin K, make sure you've thoroughly researched the implications of these choices. It's also prudent to discuss them in advance with the baby's doctor and to include them in your birthing preferences. When state law mandates such procedures, however, refusal may be a difficult option.

More Endorphins

Endorphins have carried you through this amazing, big thing you've done: birthing. And now, endorphins are your reward. The hormonal shift that takes place when the placenta leaves your body and your primal self responds to your baby's smells and pheromones deluges your system with endorphins. You may feel so ecstatic that nothing even seems real except this baby in your arms and your partner's loving touches and soft words. You may have wanted to nap at 9 centimeters, but now you're wide awake. This further supports the bonding that's taking place between you and your baby. It also strengthens the bond you feel with your partner. Everyone you see right now, you love with all the intensity of your being.

At no other time during your life, whether this is your first or fourth baby, will you feel so certain you know what to do as a parent than in these first hours following your baby's birth. This is *your* baby, and you don't need to ask anyone what to do or have your partner do an Internet search for "breastfeeding" for you. Survival of the species is imprinted in your DNA, not on the Internet or in a textbook! All those worries, doubts, and fears that come with being a parent arrive later, when your conscious brain kicks in and you start to think about why you're doing what you're doing. But for right now, the entire focus is on the *what*, and you're already doing it.

Don't be surprised, by the way, if all of a sudden that loving touch from your partner drops away and those words of wonder and joy trail off. Your partner's adrenaline has been running high all this time, and now it's gone. It's normal for your partner to want to sleep right after the birth, while you're still high. Soon enough you'll come back to earth and realize you spent all that time in labor and birthed a baby, and you'll want to sleep, too.

> ### Trusty Midwife Tips
>
> When your birth takes place at a birthing center or a hospital, staff there prepare everything you need for a birth certificate (the procedure varies among states). When you have a homebirth, your midwife will do the same. It's worthy to ask your midwife about this, though, so you know whether there's anything you have to do.

Talk to Your Baby

Your baby has been listening to the sounds of your voices for quite some time, and now he's curious to connect those sounds with what he sees, touches, and tastes. Talk to your baby! Tell him all about what an astonishing journey the two of you have had. Tell him about his siblings, his home, his grandparents, and his aunts and uncles. Babies know and remember so much more than we recognize. A number of studies have shown that young children can play with toy hospital setups and recreate the settings of their births.

It's especially important to talk with your baby, to soothe and reassure him, if things didn't turn out the way you planned. You and your partner together can help validate the experience for your baby—and for yourselves. Rather than saying, "It's okay"—because you all know it was scary and not okay at times—you may say to your baby, "We know that was scary for you, and we know you were asking for help. We got scared, too, but everything turned out fine and we're so happy you're here."

Such dialogue helps you process your own fears and emotions about what happened, too, and to recognize that you did make all the right decisions and take all the right actions for your best birth to manifest. It strengthens the bond you feel with your baby when you can share your feelings. If you doubt the power of such interaction, just look at your baby. He's calm and relaxed, yet intensely focused on you. He's listening.

The Least You Need to Know

◆ With a nonmedicated birth, a newborn is awake, alert, and curious from the moment of those first breaths.

◆ There is great benefit for both you and your baby when your baby goes right from your womb to your chest.

◆ Talking to your baby in soft, gentle tones helps him feel welcome, wanted, loved, and safe.

◆ Nearly all babies will latch onto the breast within an hour of birth, setting in motion the hormonal changes necessary in the woman's body to produce milk and the baby's body to draw nourishment from that milk.

Postpartum: What You'll Feel Like

In This Chapter

- ◆ Why does everyone get to sleep and eat but you?
- ◆ You're hormonal … again
- ◆ Let people help you
- ◆ Back to sex

For nearly a year, you've been waiting for this time. Your baby is finally in your arms, dressed in one of the cute little outfits you picked out when you first learned your pregnancy test was positive. She's so beautiful that you could sit and stare at her from now until she graduates high school.

For the first three days, you're consciously incompetent about this baby thing (even if you've done this before). You just know there's so much you don't know! But at six weeks, you're subconsciously competent. You're doing all the right things for all the right reasons, without even thinking about it.

Think of it like driving a car: teens think they know everything about driving because they've been watching adults drive all their lives. Then they get behind the wheel and something unexpected happens. They realize it's a lot more complicated than they thought, and worry about every little detail. Give them just a couple of months behind the wheel, though, and they drive like they've been doing it all their lives. Parenting your new baby is not so much different.

Welcome to the Twilight Zone

By your third postpartum day, you're living in an alternate universe where there are no nights and days. There's no schedule to your day except the one your baby imposes, and that seems totally random. You find yourself trying to choose between sleeping and eating … and often you fall asleep before you can decide. So you eat when you can squeeze it in or when you remember that you're hungry—which means you're not eating all that much.

Everyone who was so excited to come see the new baby has now gone—ostensibly so you can get your rest but also because they have to get back to their own lives and responsibilities. You're not quite sure what "getting back" even means for you; all you're getting is lonely and sleep-deprived. You may even be feeling a bit down—what people call the baby blues. You're still overjoyed to have your baby in your arms at last, but you are beginning to wonder how you'll manage. Not sleeping and not eating have this effect.

Trusty Midwife Tips

It's natural to feel a bit of an emotional letdown in the first week or so after your baby is born. There was a lot of anticipation and excitement leading up to the birth, and now that the baby is here, that's dropped off. People who call tend to ask about the baby, and you can end up feeling neglected. It was fun to be the center of attention during your pregnancy, and it's normal to miss it when it ends. You can help counter this by doing something a little special for yourself each day. Make it simple, so it doesn't get swept aside in the rush of daily activity. Maybe you sit for 10 minutes in your garden, or brew a pot of the tea you save for guests. You *are* special!

Another Hormonal Shift

At day three, you experience yet another monumental hormone shift. This shift propels your body into sustenance mode. All those breastfeeding hormones are replacing the pregnancy and birth hormones, and your body is reshaping itself once again. Any worries you may have had about whether your breasts could really sustain your baby disappear literally overnight. You wake up on that third day and holy Toledo, you've got bodacious boobs! Even if you've experienced this before, it can be a shock. Not only can you feed your own baby, but you look and feel like you could feed everyone else's baby, too. Your milk is in.

Feed Me!

And just like that, you're ravenous. Eating now takes priority over sleeping—at least, in the short term. Nice meals don't matter; you'll eat straight from the fridge. You need an extra 500 calories a day and half again as much water as you've been drinking to fuel your milk production, and you're already down a few thousand from the energy exertion of birth and not eating much in the few days following. You have some making up to do, and you're on it with a vengeance.

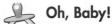 **Oh, Baby!**

It's so important to stay well hydrated when you're breastfeeding—not only because you need the fluid for your milk supply, but also because dehydration is the leading cause of breast infections (mastitis).

Did you lay in a supply of favorite foods to carry you through your birthing? If you've had a homebirth or less than a 24-hour stay at a birthing center or hospital, whatever's left of that food is still good and waiting for you, to carry you through your first day or so following the birth. If you were especially busy during your nesting time in prelabor, you may have a freezer full of foods and even complete meals that you can simply thaw, heat, and eat. When your hunger kicks in, though, any such supply will soon disappear.

It's good if you've made a list before your anticipated birth date so your partner can now go shopping to restock the cupboards. You may have different tastes and cravings now, though, so you may want to review the list or write a new one before your partner heads off to the store. If the store is close and you're feeling up to it, you may even want to go out yourself and leave your partner to be primary parent for an hour. Sometimes a brief break is remarkably restorative.

I *Love* My Baby ... May I Have Another Tissue, Please?

Day three is also when you're likely to spend the entire day feeling great and crying. The shift of having the pregnancy hormones drop and the breastfeeding hormones take over is a wild ride. No one really tells you about this; you hear and read about "being hormonal," but details are in scarce supply. Most childbirth education classes take you to crowning; often, there is little talk about what happens in the days and weeks postpartum. Most notably, no one says anything about the range of emotions—and the rapid swings between them—that are normal. Even when this information is part of your birthing education classes, it's hard to be prepared for the experience of it.

You may look at your baby and smile, then burst into tears and have no idea why. Is it love? Is it joy? Is it worry? Is it a sense of loss for the life you had before the birth, when even strangers fawned over you? It's okay—it may be all of these or none of these, but it's normal. Have another tissue. You're not being selfish or rejecting your baby … you're hormonal. Your body will adjust to this newest set of hormones in a few weeks, and you'll feel like yourself again.

> ### 🧸 Natural Woman
>
> Midwife Jenny had a couple who made the plan to cuddle in bed together for a while on the third postpartum day so they could hold each other and talk and cry as the woman's newest round of hormones took effect, anticipating that it would be a day of emotional upheaval. It was an intense bonding experience for them and helped them to understand what each was feeling about the experience of the birth, the new baby, and parenting.

A Little Help, Please

We live in a culture where often there's not much extended family nearby, and your closest relative may be at least a time zone away. The time of women coming together to see each other through birthing and the first weeks postpartum are sadly long gone. You may have a mother, aunt, sister, or friend who can come stay for a few days, which is especially helpful if you have other children at home. Make sure it's someone who you're comfortable being around. Even asking a friend or neighbor to come sit when the baby is most likely to be napping so you can get a shower or a nap yourself can be enormously helpful.

Now is when you need a little help from your family and friends—or a postpartum doula. Some couples feel guilty about paying for someone to come in and take care of things or feel that they should be able to do everything themselves. But even if your partner is able to stay home for the first few weeks or longer, it's nice to have someone who's impartial to turn to for advice and assistance. A postpartum doula can offer suggestions about breastfeeding, fix your meals, pick up groceries, and sweep your kitchen floor the same way you do.

Sometimes other people's idea of helping means taking the baby. While occasionally this may be what you want (sometimes standing in the shower until the hot water runs out feels like an extravagant luxury), mostly your baby *needs* to be with you—and what others need to do to help are tasks such as fixing meals, cleaning the house, answering the phone, and taking care of the other kids if there are any.

And you need, too, to let your priorities shift. Let "the house isn't clean like I would clean it" go. People who know and love you already know you're a domestic goddess. So what if your feet don't touch the floor in the kitchen? Nobody who comes to visit is going to stand there with a clipboard and a checklist and say, "The baby's cute, but oh my, look at that kitchen floor!" No one's looking at anything but that cute baby. So let your partner or someone else do the cleaning and housework, and let it be whatever it is. There are more important, meaningful ways for you to focus your energy—like on that oh so cute baby!

Trusty Midwife Tips

Everyone wants to know how the baby's doing. But you may not have time or be able to talk when the phone rings. Use your outgoing message to record the information about the baby. You can record updates weekly. Family and friends who call then get to hear your voice and all about life with baby—and you get to finish changing that diaper.

Everybody Loves a Baby

You're excited for all your family and friends to come meet the new baby, and they're thrilled to finally see this little bundle of joy. You could have people coming and going nearly 24 hours a day if you let them. You can't. Take a page from Mary Kaye … have your partner tell people, "I have an appointment time at 10 A.M. on Tuesday and an appointment time at 2 P.M. on Friday. Which works better for you?"

Have several people come at the same time, and keep the visit to half an hour or less. That's plenty of time for you and your partner to tell the story of the birth, let your visitors ooh and ahh over the baby, and engage in the conversation about whether the baby looks more like Mom or Dad. But it's not so long that you feel exhausted by the time everybody leaves. Most people understand and are good about this, especially if you've discussed it with them before the birth.

Pace Yourself

Many women have a tendency to do too much on postpartum days four and five (such as cleaning the kitchen floor). Almost like clockwork, you reach a point of being tired yet restless. You want to do *something*. You may even believe if only you were doing more, you could then sleep. This is false logic, but it comes from a hormonal base—so it makes perfect sense to you at the time.

Your entire world, it seems, is breasts and baby, and you want to do more—to return to *yourself*. This *is* yourself, at least for the next six to eight weeks. It's not only okay but desirable to let yourself be the mom and for your sole focus to be your baby. Much of your restlessness comes from being everything to everyone before the birth; the calm of giving all of you to your new baby can be unsettling.

Cramping and bleeding, which tend to subside by the fourth postpartum day, will escalate again if you push yourself to do more. Your body will rise to the occasion, but if you keep it up, at six weeks—almost to the hour of birth—you'll crash and feel worse than you did on day two. If you'll just give yourself these five days (and better yet, take ten), then you'll be fine at six weeks. If you cheat them, you'll pay.

Two Weeks: A Milestone

If you get to the two-week mark without overdoing it, congratulations! You're an exception, and by taking it easy you've done the very best for yourself and your baby that's possible, even if it doesn't feel that way to you. If you're still taking care of yourself and letting others help you in the ways that they're able to help at two weeks, you'll likely continue.

This doesn't mean that things suddenly get easy. You're still making deals with yourself to get through the day. There's a light at the end of the tunnel that you can recognize as the glimmer of your new normal life, but that train's not in the station quite yet. It really is about six weeks before you feel confident about what you're doing. It's good to know this, because it takes the pressure off trying to be there now.

Baby Blues ... or Postpartum Depression?

Nearly all women experience periods of feeling down, alone, and incapable of meeting what seem to be the disproportionately enormous needs of a tiny being. These feelings are very normal and arise from a combination of hormones, the changes in your lifestyle the new baby brings, not enough to eat to sustain your own energy, and sleep deprivation from napping your way through each day and night. (Sleeping and eating are even a bigger deal than you think.) When these feelings continue for more than a few days or even into weeks, or you feel so overwhelmed that you can't function, you're dealing with more than the baby blues.

Trusty Midwife Tips

An unsatisfactory birth experience can set postpartum depression in motion. Even when your birthing turns out differently than you expected, it's important to give yourself permission to know that you did the best you could to make your best birth possible. When you feel your birth was hijacked, there's a lot of postpartum doubt. When you participate in each decision along the course of your birth, there's no "coulda woulda shoulda" to plague you. Say out loud to yourself, "I made my best birth possible." Believe it. It's true.

Postpartum depression is a serious condition that can even be a psychotic break (a complete loss of connection with reality). It's somewhat insidious because we have such a cultural stigma attached to it that even (or especially) new mothers don't want to acknowledge its symptoms and effects. You've crossed into depression when you can't pull yourself out of your feelings. These are key red flags:

♦ You feel life is not worth living.

♦ You look at your partner with resentment, anger, or even hatred because your partner "gets" to go to work and you "have" to stay home with the baby.

♦ You haven't showered for days … and you don't notice or don't care.

♦ You feel no connection to your baby or desire to respond to your baby's cries and needs.

♦ The idea of having to drag yourself through one more day is completely overwhelming.

If you have any of these feelings, *talk to someone.* Talk to your partner. Call your midwife or doctor. Talk to your mother, your sister, or your best friend. Asking for help is really hard for many people. We have a cultural expectation that women should be able to do it all—with a smile. We can't! And we shouldn't feel that we can. But we're afraid to share fears, doubts, and feelings—often even with our partners—because we don't want to be viewed as crazy or incompetent. Our society also attaches a lot of expectations on motherhood, many of which are unrealistic but persist nonetheless.

Causes and Treatments

The causes of postpartum depression are unclear. The prevailing theory is that the sudden absence of all those pregnancy and birthing hormones—which drop immediately after birth—triggers an imbalance among the biochemicals in the brain that regulate mood and emotion. Because the cause of postpartum depression is biochemical, you cannot "will" yourself to feel better.

Natural Woman

American actress Brooke Shields focused public attention on postpartum depression with her 2005 book, *Down Came the Rain: My Journey Through Postpartum Depression* (NY: Hyperion). Shields continues to appear on talk shows to discuss her experiences and spoke out in support of federal legislation to provide funding for postpartum depression research and treatment programs. She stresses the need to lift the stigma that accompanies postpartum depression so women will seek care when they have symptoms.

Doing what you can to reduce the stress in your daily life seems to help many women who have postpartum depression. Involve family members and friends as your "support crew" to help out with everyday tasks and even taking care of your baby for short periods of time so you can have some time to yourself. Try to get more sleep—easier said than done with a new baby, we know, but sleep is remarkably restorative.

Physical activity, such as walking, releases endorphins (remember those from birthing?). It may also help your body more quickly return to its normal biochemical balance. Your doctor may recommend treatment with antidepressant medications, which work by rebalancing brain chemicals. How long you may need to take them will depend on your symptoms.

Compounding Factors

You can't be your best self when you only sleep 2 or 3 out of every 24 hours. But things are not always going to be this way. Indeed, you'll be stunned at how quickly you leave this time behind. When your baby is suddenly that teenager getting behind the wheel, you may even long for a return to these days! If something's not working for you, don't do it. There are many ways to accomplish the same things, and you need to feel free to find what works for you.

You may have to put much of this in place yourself, which isn't right or fair but is sometimes how it ends up. We don't have, as a standard, the kinds of support networks in place that women with new babies need. You may have a midwife or a doctor who organizes support groups and has a three- or five-day follow-up to see how you're doing. But the conventional model pretty much leaves you on your own until your two-week postpartum visit. Again, we say, ***talk to someone.*** At the very least, you'll have yet something else to look back on and laugh about. And at the very best, you may save yourself a lot of emotional trauma. Chances are, the very same thing is going on in households all across the country. It's such a relief to find out you're not the only one and to learn how others are dealing with the same things.

> **Trusty Midwife Tips**
>
> Be kind to yourself! You couldn't do *everything* before your baby was born, and you can't do *everything* now. You need others to pitch in, and even do a little extra, with household chores and daily tasks.

Especially make the effort to share your feelings with your partner, even when it's hard. Be aware that the truth may shoot out of you in harsh and unexpected ways—a function of sleep deprivation and hormones. But once things are out there, you can talk through them. The transition can be particularly rough when yours is a household where you do everything. Your partner truly may not know what needs to be done around the house, as irrational as this sounds. When you're the one doing everything, who's going to get in the way of that?

It's often helpful to develop "postpartum preferences," too, before the birth. You can establish what you'd like for your partner to take over for you and also uncover any uncertainties your partner may feel about doing so. Insecurity about competence is a two-way street. You may decide the best option is to have someone come stay for a few weeks, such as your mom or a sister, to keep the peace regarding tasks no one wants to take on. And you may need to let go of your own expectations of how things get done and agree to accept whatever it looks like when someone else steps in. You'll be back at the helm sooner than you think. All these days that feel like they'll never end are temporary—it just doesn't feel like that while you're living it.

The Return of Real Life (SEX)

One day you'll look at your partner coming up the walk after work, and you'll want to head right for the bedroom. You've ovulated, and your body is saying, "Hey, let's make another baby!" Of course, what this sounds like to you right now is, "Hey, let's have sex!"

Your partner may be overjoyed or apprehensive … or both. Sex changes forever after a baby, and both of you know this. You just may not know what that means and whether it's good or bad. You may have worries about how you'll fit together now and how things will go with your breasts full of milk.

Your perineum takes time to heal, even if only from the stretching required to let your baby out—and of course if you had an episiotomy or a tear, it takes longer to feel ready. The bigger factor in your return to sex, however, comes back to those hormones. Yep, once again your hormones are running the show. And here's the typical script: your milk comes in, prolactin skyrockets, and estrogen plummets. Prolactin makes you crave that double-D bra with two-inch straps and drop-down cups, not the latest lacey delight from Victoria's Secret. That's estrogen's job, and frequent nursing keeps your estrogen in the basement. You have less than no desire to have sex or even think about it.

As the baby's feedings become further apart, estrogen starts to climb up a little. Then comes the evening when you look at each other and say, "We've gotta get out of here!" So, you get a sitter, put on some real clothes, and go to the movies. You're gone two hours, and it's a lot of fun to be alone together. So you decide to have a quick meal, just the two of you, in an adult setting (which means anywhere you don't place your order at a drive-through window). And it's nice to sit and eat slowly enough to identify your food and even talk at the same time.

The usual time of your baby's feeding slips by. You notice it because your breasts are feeling uncomfortably full, but there are a few bottles of breast milk in the fridge at home—so your baby's needs are covered. A quick call home reassures that all is quiet. So you decide you can ignore your discomfort for another hour or so, and you extend your evening out. It feels almost like a date.

The pressure in your breasts subdues prolactin, and estrogen creeps farther out of the basement. More importantly, this one night has set in motion a cascade of events in your body that result in ovulation: after more than a year, you've finally released another egg. This usually occurs somewhere around six months postpartum (although it can happen as early as six weeks postpartum). Your partner suddenly looks like the sexiest man on earth, and you can't have sex with him fast enough (or enough, period). This is the surest sign that you've ovulated, no matter what else is happening (or not happening, like a menstrual period) in your body.

You also might make another baby well before you're ready to do so: you're again fertile although you're still breastfeeding your baby. The message here is not to hold off on sex but to use birth control if you're not ready for another baby. Sex gives back to you and your partner an important intimacy in your relationship; just be sure that's the only thing it gives you until you're ready.

Trusty Midwife Tips

Talk with your midwife or doctor about contraception options that will not interfere with breastfeeding.

Your Path Is Unique

One of the most surprising discoveries you may make during the postpartum period is that you're not going to be like what you read in Chapter 2 of whatever books you bought. You're going to find your own way. You'll talk to other moms who have similar experiences, and that's affirming. It's easy to feel really isolated because you've been living only in your own world, so once you can get out and about, you begin to realize there are others with whom you can talk. And today, you can turn to online forums and blogs for support so you don't even have to leave the house if you don't want to (although it is good for you to get out once in a while). You can talk to anybody, any time, for immediate encouragement and support.

The Least You Need to Know

- It's hard to feel sane when you don't sleep or eat enough, but this won't last forever.

- When others step in to help, you need to step out of the way and let them do it; they won't do things like you do, but they'll do them well enough.

- It's normal to feel the "baby blues" every now and again, but it's not normal to feel that way all the time. It helps to be able to share your feelings, worries, and fears with someone you trust.

- If you have signs and symptoms of postpartum depression, talk to your doctor or midwife.

- Although the hormones that support breastfeeding suppress the hormones that allow ovulation, breastfeeding is *not* a form of contraception!

Chapter 23

Breastfeeding, of Course

In This Chapter

♦ The instinctive drive to root, latch, and suck

♦ It's not just about the nipple

♦ Perfect for your baby's changing needs

♦ Diaper duty

You've done all the work to have a healthy pregnancy and prepare for a natural birth—so breastfeeding your new baby is the next natural step. Your breast milk is the healthiest nutrition you can give to your newborn— the absolute perfect meal. At first, breastfeeding takes your full concentration and effort. By five weeks, however, you'll easily breastfeed your baby wherever and whenever.

There's widespread agreement that breast milk is the ideal nutritional balance for a baby from birth to two years of age or longer, although cultural norms far more than any other factor tend to influence the length of time women breastfeed their babies. Breastfeeding also nurtures a close bond between mother and baby; your breast and your baby's mouth are aligned for perfect contact with each other when you hold your baby close to you. He can feel the rhythm of your heartbeat and your breathing when snuggled in at your breast, which is greatly comforting. These are the sensations he's known all his life.

It's Not That Complicated ... Really!

To look at the wall of books at the bookstore, you'd think breastfeeding must be really complicated. It's really very simple, though. Your baby already has a rooting and sucking reflex—all those seemingly uncoordinated "baby bird" head bobs she's doing while on your chest are designed to help her find your breast. All you have to do is teach her where to root and what to suck.

The root-latch-suck reflex reaches its peak 20 to 30 minutes after birth; the baby has an impossible-to-ignore urge to put something in its mouth. The baby acts quite frantic in its efforts to find the breast during this window. Such an urge is not again so strong until 24 hours later, although the baby will still nurse in between. It became a practice in medical births in the 1960s to give the baby glucose solution (sugar water) or plain water by bottle to quell what appeared to be the baby's hunger. However, we now know that it's probably not hunger that drives this reflex so much as the survival instinct to find the food source. And we also now know that giving glucose solution or water in this way can interfere with the baby's interest in latching at the breast.

> **Natural Woman**
>
> Swedish physician Lennart Righard, M.D., and midwife Margaret Alade conducted a study published in 1990 that included an astonishing short video showing a newborn, left on its own on its mother's thighs after a natural, nonmedicated birth, following its mother's linea nigra (the dark line that runs from the pubis to the belly button), to pull and push its way to his mother's breast apparently drawn by the contrast of the dark areola against the lighter color of the breast. Both mother and infant were awake, alert, and calm. The newborn's determined journey took less than six minutes; the phenomenon is called self-attachment.

Belly to Belly: Helping Your Baby Latch

Try this: look straight ahead, keeping your chin forward. Swallow. Can you do it? Duh—of course. Now turn your head as far to one side as you can, touching your chin to your shoulder if possible. Swallow. Can you do it? Not so easy, is it? If you're holding your baby in your arms and she's gazing lovingly into your eyes, it's a beautiful bonding moment—but she can't nurse from there. She can't latch without cranking her head until her chin's on her shoulder, and even if she can latch, she won't be able to swallow—just like you couldn't very well when you turned your head.

When you look down at your baby when she's ready to nurse, you should see her ear. This tells you she's aligned with your breast in such a way that she doesn't have to turn her head to suck and swallow. Next, her mouth needs to be even with your nipple line, so all she has to do is open her mouth and your nipple will just about fall right in. All it takes are a few of those baby-bird bobs and she's on.

You can use pillows to support your arm as you hold your baby, which lets you relax your elbow and shoulder. At first you'll feel some tension in your arms because they're not used to being held in this position, but that will go away the more you do it. Pillows also put, and keep, your baby in just the right position to easily find your breast. Special pillows made for nursing are just the right height, length, and firmness. Or you can use combinations of pillows that you already have. One bed pillow is not usually high enough, although two may be too high. You'll want to experiment to find the right mix. It's good to keep pillows everywhere you may be when your baby wants to breastfeed so you can always be comfortable and relaxed.

Patience and Relaxation are Key

When your baby is new to breastfeeding, it may take her five minutes or longer to latch and begin nursing. This is normal, so get yourself settled and comfortable so you don't feel rushed or pressured. With your baby at your belly and her face to your chest, pick up your entire breast, from the chest wall, and use your nipple to tickle your baby's cheek. Talk or sing to her; this helps draw her attention to you and also helps you to relax.

> **Trusty Midwife Tips**
>
> Some babies take to the breast right away, and others seem to not know quite what to do. There are lots of tips and techniques to encourage your baby by following her cues. A lactation consultant can observe what happens when you put your baby to your breast, and then offer specific suggestions and show you how to do them. It's important to stay calm and relaxed, which helps both you and your baby.

Your baby will turn and open her mouth, often in a rather casual way at first. Do this several times until she gets a frantic, "Where is it?" kind of bobbing thing going with a big, open mouth. Put your hand against the back of your baby's head and gently push her right into your nipple. If you're too slow, her mouth will close but not on your breast. It takes practice, so be calm and patient. Your baby won't starve while you're figuring out just how to get the right move going with her head. If she starts to fuss, this is good. She's hungry and eager to nurse.

Your baby should latch at the areola, so when she sucks she pulls the nipple nearly to the back of her throat. This is a very strong pull; it surprises most moms at first, even if they've nursed other babies. The milk ducts are between the areola and the nipple, so about one third to half the areola should be in your baby's mouth—but you should still see some areola around her mouth. Your nipple has several openings for milk to come out, so the milk comes out in a spray, not a stream.

When it's time to release your baby from your breast to switch her to the other side, wet your finger and slide it into her mouth to break the seal. If you just pull your nipple out of her mouth, you'll do so only once! (Ouch!) Don't be shocked at the appearance of your nipple when it first leaves your baby's mouth after she's been breastfeeding, which is likely to look kind of flattened and elongated; it'll come back to its normal shape and size shortly.

> **Natural Woman**
>
> At the time of birth, a baby's stomach is barely the size of a marble. It doesn't take much to fill it. To give your baby the nutrition she needs, your breasts contain thick fluid called colostrum that's extraordinarily high in sugars and other vital nutrients your baby needs after the intense work of being born. Taking colostrum is a lot like sucking honey from a straw, which strengthens your baby's latching and sucking. This, too, is a survival mechanism.

Should You "Toughen" Your Nipples?

It's really difficult to simulate the effect of nursing, no matter what some books tell you about roughing up your nipples with a towel or something such. Toughening up your nipples is not really the issue, although many women new to breastfeeding experience sore nipples. The part that's being stretched is the *length* of the nipple, from its stem area just above the areola. It takes about 10 to 14 days for your nipple to be in the proper shape and condition for breastfeeding, which is one reason why things seem to magically get better at the two-week mark.

During those two weeks, you can use an herbal salve or balm, such as Purple Thistle Tea Company's Lickety-Split Healing Balm (available through midwife Jenny's website, www.tubsntea.com) or similar products available at health food stores. Many products promoted for breast care aim to keep the nipple area moist, but moisture isn't really the issue. Cracks and splits develop under the new pressures being applied to the nipple, and these need to heal. Herbal teas for nursing may also help increase your milk supply if you need it.

When you're considering what products to use (there are many on the market), pay attention to whether you need to wash off the product before breastfeeding. This may exacerbate your discomfort and delay healing. Balms made with food-grade ingredients can stay on, even when your baby nurses. The need to wash off a product may defeat the purpose of using it. It's possible to have a sensitivity to products, too, notably lanolin.

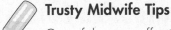

Trusty Midwife Tips

One of the most effective ways to prevent sore nipples is to rinse or gently wipe them with warm water and then let them air-dry after breastfeeding. If you leak milk between feedings, use absorbent pads or blot the milk from your breasts with a soft, absorbent cloth.

Stick With It

You do need to keep breastfeeding even with sore and chapped nipples. Some women find nursing shields to be helpful for protecting the nipples somewhat. Nursing shields are also useful if you have naturally small or inverted nipples. This is something you can assess at about 37 weeks so you're prepared by the time your baby's born. It's easy to do: if you put an ice cube on your nipple, does it stand up tall? If so, it's likely to be easy for your baby to latch and suck.

Your baby needs to feel your nipple on the roof of his mouth because this is what makes him clamp down and suck. If you are unsure about whether your nipples will let your baby do this, have a lactation consultant, midwife, or labor nurse take a look before you start labor. A few things can be done to make your nipples bigger; a lactation consultant can show these to you and help you figure out the best options for your personal situation. You may need a nipple shield, although most women do not.

As long as your baby is gaining weight and growing and you're getting lots of wet and poopy diapers, she's getting enough to eat even if you worry that she's not. Your midwife, a doula, or a lactation consultant can come to your home to help you refine your techniques so breastfeeding becomes smooth and enjoyable for both you and your baby.

Many babies like to fall asleep at the breast—and moms like it, too, for the sense of closeness it establishes. It's fine to indulge this for a short time; the bonding aspect of it is also important. But babies do best when they nurse until they're full and are then removed from the breast. Otherwise, they may partly wake up, suck a little, and fall back asleep. You'll feel like all you ever do is breastfeed—because that *is* all you're doing! This also extends the time your nipples are sore.

When You Can't Breastfeed

Sometimes, breastfeeding just doesn't work out. When this is the case, your baby's provider will recommend an infant formula and give you guidelines for making sure she gets enough nutrition. If you formula-feed, always hold your baby when feeding her. This fosters bonding, which is crucial for your baby's emotional security.

Natural Woman

Healthy People 2010, the American health improvement initiative, establishes a goal of 75 percent of women breastfeeding their babies immediately following birth, and 50 percent still breastfeeding at six months. However, major health organizations recommend all women exclusively breastfeed their babies for six months, unless there are health reasons for not breastfeeding.

Your Milk: The Perfect Baby Formula

Your breasts contain colostrum—the ultimate "high octane" natural food—for the first three days. Its thickness is just right for the infant's tiny stomach. Your baby may nurse for only five minutes and then fall asleep; however, the colostrum is enough to take the edge off. She may want to do this every hour, though! Frequent nursing assures that your baby will receive enough nutrition and tells your pituitary gland to make milk.

Frequent nursings in the first few days may bring your milk in early. It also keeps your baby's digestive tract moving, helping clear out all that tarry meconium poop. If your baby nurses longer than five minutes or so in the first three days, however, she's mostly doing non-nutritive nursing because her tiny tummy can't hold very much. Being at your breast makes her feel safe and loved, and she likes it.

In addition to being the perfect nutrition for your newborn, your colostrum carries a wallop of antibodies into your baby's body every time she nurses. This helps protect her against infection while her immune system is maturing; many immunologists believe colostrum sets up the baby's immunity for life. Despite the abundance of sophisticated technology available today, scientists still do not know the precise composition of colostrum—nor have they been able to replicate it in a laboratory.

The Real Deal

Around the end of day two or the start of day three, depending on how strongly your baby sucks, your milk comes in. (If you had an epidural, your milk's arrival is typically delayed by however long the epidural was in.) Until now, your baby has been sucking at nice, soft breasts. She has had to work to extract the colostrum, of course, but it has been a pleasant kind of work.

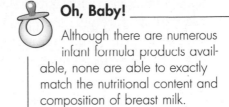

Oh, Baby!

Although there are numerous infant formula products available, none are able to exactly match the nutritional content and composition of breast milk.

Day three brings a shock: your breasts are now more like overinflated beach balls, and the milk they contain is thin. Don't be surprised if your baby pulls off your breast as soon as that milk hits the back of her throat. Just help her get back on; she'll get the hang of it. Watch her jaw move, listen for sounds, watch and feel for her to swallow. The first few times having real milk, your baby gets so satiated it's like she's "milk-drunk"—and she'll probably fall asleep at your breast.

On day three, your baby's stomach is about the size of a shooter marble—not quite an inch in diameter although triple its size on day one. The thin milk isn't as nutritionally dense as the colostrum, so she needs more of it to meet her needs. Her stomach grows so it can hold more, and by day 10 her stomach is about the size of a golf ball. This is pretty substantial for her, even though it still sounds small. She may hold enough to feel comfortable for three hours now.

Oh, Baby!

You'll find that some of your favorite foods don't agree with your baby. Cabbage, broccoli, chocolate (sorry!), and onions are highest on the list of troublemakers. Even if you've been eating these foods all your life, they're new to your baby and her developing digestive system. It's a good idea to avoid these foods while you're breastfeeding. Some indications that your diet is upsetting your baby's system include excessive fussiness, gas, and smelly poops. A lactation consultant, your midwife, or your doctor can help you figure this out.

Is Your Baby Getting Enough?

Your baby doesn't yet know the correlation between feeling hungry and her rooting and sucking behaviors, so she's learning this. Babies tend to start sleeping a little longer when the milk comes in because they're finally full. Your baby should eat when she's hungry; you'll learn her patterns soon enough. If she has a short feed, she'll want to eat again sooner. If she has a long feed, she may sleep for three hours.

More babies tend toward "nipping and napping" in the first stages of real breast milk because they get so full so fast that they do fall asleep on the nipple. Using the wet finger to break the seal, remove your baby from your breast. If she awakens and tries frantically to relatch, wait one minute. If she's still fussy, let her nurse some more—she's not full. If she falls asleep, she's had her fill.

By day 10, your baby's stomach is the size of a golf ball or ping-pong ball, and she's ready for a growth spurt. She's going to eat all the time for about a day, and this is normal. Then she'll be back to a normal eating pattern, which will be more than she was taking before but not as much as during her growth spurt. Over those next couple days, though, you're going to have a lot more milk than the baby will consume. This is a great time to pump that extra milk so you can refrigerate or freeze it.

> **Trusty Midwife Tips** _____
>
> There are lots of breast pumps on the market—manual, electric, and battery. What matters most is to choose one that's comfortable and easy for you to use. It's best to pump from full breasts rather than after your baby has nursed for a while. Rotate your stored milk stock and use your oldest first (yes, you have to date it!). You can store breast milk in the refrigerator for 24 hours or in the freezer for up to three months. It's best to use it fairly quickly, though, because your breast milk also changes as your baby grows.

Poop

A good gauge for whether your baby is getting enough to eat is whether she's pooping and peeing. This can be hard to tell with current disposable diapers because they contain crystals that absorb the pee. The diaper may feel dry, so you have to feel for the bulge of the now saturated crystals and the heaviness of the diaper. Peeing is the best measure that your baby is getting enough fluid, so you want to be seeing lots of wet diapers. Because breast milk is nature's design for your baby, it provides the perfect balance of water and nutrients—a balance that changes as your baby grows and her needs change. Pretty cool to have the perfect sustenance right there on your chest!

Your baby's first bowel movements are to push out the meconium—the thick, tar-like substance intended to protect her intestines while she's floating in amniotic fluid. After birth, she needs her intestines to function, so she has to expel all that meconium. It's the most defiant stuff to get off your baby, off you, and out of cloth diapers! Even if you're planning to use cloth diapers, consider using disposable diapers for the first three days. And before you put that first diaper on your baby (as well as for every diaper change during the meconium stage), grease up every part of your baby's skin that will be under the diaper. You can use just olive oil or an unscented massage oil. Get in all the nooks and crannies. The oil will keep the meconium from sticking to the skin, letting you wipe it off with three or four baby wipes.

Your baby's stools will become normal when your breast milk comes in and she's nursing regularly. They look kind of like watery, mustard-colored cottage cheese. (Now you'll probably never eat mustard or cottage cheese again!) It's true that breast milk stools have no foul odor. They're consistently soft in texture but not runny and clean easily from your baby's skin as well as from cloth diapers.

Breastfed babies tend to poop more often than formula-fed babies, although there is less volume. Breast milk is the perfect match for your baby's digestive system, so she uses nearly all of it. It's only if your baby's pooping schedule changes that you should pay attention. (Except, that is, at day 10, when she has her growth spurt. Everything gets disturbed then, including her pooping schedule. She may not poop for several days; it's as though her entire body resets and uses every calorie.)

A Lifelong Foundation

Breastfeeding benefits your baby now as well as throughout life. You're laying a foundation not only for nutrition but also for your baby to feel cherished, wanted, and important. When you're nursing, your baby is the center of your attention. You can't really do much else when your baby's at your breast—and why would you want to, when you can just sit with this beautiful creation? It's simply not possible to hold, snuggle, and love a baby too much; there's no such thing as spoiling your newborn. Babies need as much close contact with their parents as they can get. And you need this connection, too. Love flows in both directions.

Natural Woman _____

A recent large-scale study showed that children who were breastfed as babies had IQs an average of five points higher than children who were not breastfed as infants. In their analysis, the researchers determined that 60 percent of the increased IQ—3.2 points—was the direct result of breast milk's nutritional composition. The researchers attributed the remaining 40 percent to the effects of bonding between mother and infant through the process of breastfeeding.

The Least You Need to Know

◆ Your baby has an intense drive to latch and suck about 20 to 30 minutes after birth; this intensity does not return for another 24 hours.

◆ The colostrum your breasts contain for the first three days after birth is densely nutritious and also contains antibodies to boost your baby's developing immune system.

◆ Breast milk is the ideal food for your baby, changing to meet her needs as she grows and develops.

◆ The close physical contact between you and your baby that occurs with breast-feeding establishes a lifelong foundation of love and security for your baby.

Chapter 24

You'd Do It All Again

In This Chapter

- The power of birth's energy
- No secrets
- A midwife's initiation
- A matter of trust
- Of art and creativity

When the energy of natural birth touches you, it changes you for life. All you want to do is keep touching it! Woman after woman tells midwife Jenny, "I can't believe it's over … I can't wait to do it again!" even as she's still sitting in the birthing tub, her newborn snuggled on her chest. What better endorsement, what better motivation for choosing a natural birth in the first place than going into it already knowing you'd choose it again?

The power of this energy has touched the lives of women for millennia, passing from one generation to the next through all fashions of story-telling and shared experiences. It draws together, in a circle of ancient wisdom, all who give birth and all who witness birth. How empowering, how liberating, how joyful the idea that you can create for yourself a birth story that you want to tell for the rest of your life.

With Woman

Midwives live in the flow of birth's energy every day. Each birth is unique and special to the woman giving birth, her partner, and her family. There's something about a midwife that makes it seem as though things are possible when she's present that otherwise could not or would not happen.

"I don't do it for them, I just get to be there when they do it," says midwife Jenny. "I don't make births happen, or create the experiences a woman has of birth. That's what she does. What I do get to do is watch a woman realize she can do anything. She's trusted her body, and now there are no limits."

Jenny jokes that midwifery is the second-oldest profession for women, and midwives are still out on the fringe. The humor is bittersweet; there is an odd sense of competitiveness and control in our contemporary society surrounding what should be a simple and straightforward role of supporting women to empower themselves. Yet, letting go and going with the flow is the ultimate control—and nothing teaches you that like birth.

> **Trusty Midwife Tips**
>
> Once you stand in the energy of natural birth, you're changed forever. It informs every creative act you'll experience for the rest of your life. And when you're planning a natural birth, it's a completely different energy for your baby. Your baby knows this!

"I do wish for every woman to enjoy her birth, to figure out how to claim and hold her own space," Jenny says. "I want to hear every woman say she can hardly wait to be in labor again, to feel those feelings. This is so opposite what we're taught to expect about birth in our culture but there it is, right there in front of me, every day."

The Secret

Many women, when they first start hearing about natural birth, believe there has to be some sort of secret no one has let them in on. Especially when they hear about how wonderful the midwife was; how transforming it was to get into the birthing tub; and how it was possible to enter such a deep trance that the outside world simply disappears. Other women know something; midwives know something; *somebody* knows something. If you could only discover what this "something" is, then you, too, could have the most amazing—even orgasmic—birth.

The secret is, there are no secrets. Women who have natural births talk about their experiences all the time—openly, often, and in great detail. Most will answer any questions you ask; there's no keeping them from talking. They want to tell you *everything.* They attempt to describe with words the deepest and most intimate of emotions and sensations, and when you hear their stories, you want what they have. Clearly, their birth experiences live with them now, in the present—not only as memories.

Women truly are strong. Everything you are as a woman is designed to bring forth new life. Not that birth is your only purpose in life, but that birth can be one of the fullest expressions and experiences of yourself. And the birth experience you choose is only the beginning, helping to inform your first experiences of motherhood and shaping your path as a mother.

Trust Yourself

You have to do what you have to do to get to a place where you trust yourself. When you set forth on this path, it's often astonishing to discover just what you *can* do. This is as true in life as it is in birth, and if birth is the step to get there, great! A natural birth does change you, and it changes you for the better. You did this, you flew in the light of an ancient womanly tradition, and you did it well. You have felt—to the deepest core of your being, and in every cell of your body—the power of creation. It is encoded within you, and your baby's arrival into the world is your proof. You can now do and be *anything;* what could possibly stop you?

It's important to have a competent, knowledgeable, qualified professional attending your birth—not because you need her help to birth your baby, but because you can trust her to watch everything that needs watching so you can fully enter your birth experience. You know she's there, just like a spotter is present for a gymnast. It's a "just-in-case" presence, not a "what-if" presence. (The "what-ifs" will drive you crazy, but "just in case" makes sense.)

Natural Woman

"Birth is not only about making babies. It's about making mothers—strong, competent, capable mothers who trust themselves and believe in their inner strength."

Barbara Katz Rothman (1948–), American sociologist and author

"Just in case" says your midwife will catch the small stuff, keeping your path clear so all you need to do is focus on working with your body's efforts. She makes sure the birthing tub temperature is exactly right for you and offers words of encouragement that you're doing everything exactly right. She answers your questions and assures you things are going just as they should. But mostly, she's just there—and when she's doing her best for you, you seldom even notice her presence.

Natural Woman

More mothers than not have more than one child, but so far none have topped the eighteenth-century wife of Russian peasant Feodor Vassilyev (whose name, unfortunately, did not survive recordkeeping). The *Guinness Book of World Records* reports that in the 40 years between 1725 and 1765, the couple's 27 pregnancies produced 69 babies, including 4 sets of quadruplets, 7 sets of triplets, and 16 pairs of twins.

Catching Babies

When Jenny first thought she wanted to become a midwife, she volunteered at a midwifery clinic so she could see what it was all about. Late one night, a staff midwife grabbed her arm and took her into a birthing room and sat her on a bed between a laboring woman's legs. A little banana-like wedge of the baby's head was showing. Jenny was stunned; she was only supposed to be there to watch, not to actually do anything.

While her brain was busy telling her all the reasons she couldn't be doing what she was doing, Jenny's hands reached forward to support that little head as it was emerging. "The mother was sweaty, had that inward-focused look of concentration on her face that I would come to know as the power of birth," Jenny says. "And I would come to know that it didn't really matter who sat down on the bed. I still say I didn't do a thing. I was just placed in front of a baby coming out of a woman. It just happened to come out in my hands. Because I was there, I could catch babies. The mother sat up to take her baby, and that was it." From that day on, Jenny knew she wanted to stand witness to that awesome, creative joy for any woman who asked her.

Today, as a full-time midwife, Jenny focuses on guiding parents through their birthing experiences. She's not there to catch the baby but rather to educate couples to help them make the decisions they need to make. "I'm reminding women that they already know how to do this, putting them back in touch with that inner wisdom, the birthing goddess, whatever you want to call it," Jenny says. "Every birthing woman should have the experience of feeling her baby pushing off her rib cage to push itself down, and then feel the kicking when the baby can't reach the rib cage any more."

Birth, the Greatest Story Ever Written

Midwife Jenny has attended hundreds of births and sees the full range of emotions and reactions as parents finally greet the new baby. "I see relief, joy, satisfaction, and anxiety until the baby makes noises to let everybody know he's okay, and I do get to see that starry look of love when the mother looks for her partner's face as she holds her new baby to her chest," Jenny says. "It's an unbelievably amazing moment, *every* time."

Each birth is a unique and powerful story; no one story is more significant than another. Some, however, get a lot more press. Singer Erykah Badu tweeted the 2009 story of her daughter's homebirth on Twitter, according to babiesonline.com. Erykah gave birth without medications after a five-hour labor.

Actress Naomi Watts also enjoys motherhood redux, telling *People* magazine after her second son's birth in late 2008, "There is much less fear this time. You are much more old-hand at it." So much so that the celebrity website WhyFame.com quotes her as saying, "I love babies. I look at this little baby and, even after quite an intense birth—they say you have amnesia, as women—I would go a third. It would be nice to have a girl."

> **Trusty Midwife Tips**
>
> Consider a natural birth because it's the right thing for you, your baby, and your partner. Do it because you figured out this is what you want, based on accurate information on both sides—not because someone else did it or wants you to do it. The goal is to have mothers and babies who are not only healthier but happier with their birthing experiences.

Pop star Usher is among the celeb dads giving the other side of the story, telling *MTV News* following the birth of his second son in late 2008, "I would never miss any of my children being born. It's an incredible experience. Any person who has children can definitely agree with me when I say it is by far one of the greatest experiences of life. I'm very happy."

From the Waterfall to the Lighthouse

Australian actress Nicole Kidman has brought a number of memorable characters to life in her illustrious career. Every now and then, though, the real drama that takes place is so amazing, it couldn't be scripted. Such was the case when Kidman was filming the epic *Australia* (released in 2008), suitably, in the Australian outback. While in the remote town of Kununurra, Kidman and six other women from the cast and crew sought respite from the mostly arid environment by swimming in the area's several waterfalls.

No one thought much of it beyond the refreshing coolness of the water amid the breath-taking scenery—until Kidman realized that she and husband Keith Urban were expecting a baby. Within days, the other six women reported that they, too, were pregnant. Kidman said in an interview that she'd believed she'd never become pregnant. "But it happened on this movie," she's quoted as saying. "There is something up there in the Kununurra water." Through her creative effort as an artist, and a little help perhaps from the waters, Kidman achieved the personal creativity she thought she would never have.

Kidman bridges time and art form to share a creative bond with famed novelist Virginia Woolf, whom Kidman portrayed in the 2002 film *The Hours.* Kidman won a Golden Globe Award and the Academy Award for Best Actress for the role. Woolf approached the duality of creativity from the other direction in her 1927 novel, *To the Lighthouse.* In this masterful work, Woolf examines what it means to be an artist, and her novel's heroine, Mrs. Ramsay—the mother of eight—personifies the beauty, elegance, and fecundity of the creative home life. It takes a lot of energy to make a home and tend to your family, as you're discovering now! No doubt this passage from the novel could describe *you* and so wonderfully captures how you feel at the end of a day and how worth it motherhood is ... even when you're tired:

> **Natural Woman**
>
> Of the seven women who conceived after swimming in the Kununurra waterfalls, six birthed daughters—including award-winning actress Nicole Kidman, who named her daughter Sunday Rose after an Australian artist whose work she admires.

"Immediately, Mrs. Ramsay seemed to fold herself together, one petal closed in another, and the whole fabric fell in exhaustion upon itself, so that she had only strength enough to move her finger, in exquisite abandonment to exhaustion, across the page of Grimm's fairy story, while there throbbed through her, like the pulse in a spring which has expanded to its full width and now gently ceases to beat, the rapture of successful creation."

It is an amazing thing to look at this child of your creation, who is at once a part of you and yet apart from you, an individual with personality and preferences not necessarily what you imagined them to be. It's only natural to want to engage in this creativity again (and again!) to experience the wonder of this art of life.

> **Natural Woman**
>
> *Time* magazine, in a review of Julia Roberts's movie *Duplicity,* quotes Roberts as saying that working brings form into the "shapeless blob of happy chaos" that is motherhood. The review's writer, Mary Pols, resonates so much to this idea that she says she'd "be willing to give [Roberts the] $10 [price of admission] just for summing up the working mother's perspective so nicely."

Full Circle

Real life becomes art in the Pulitzer Prize–winning *A Midwife's Tale: The Life of Martha Ballard Based on Her Diary, 1785–1812*, by noted American historian Laurel Thatcher Ulrich. Ballard was a midwife in New England, in what would become the state of Maine. The book was also produced as a PBS film in PBS's The *American Experience* series.

Ulrich's impressive work used Martha Ballard's writings about birthing and other matters as a lens through which to examine the roles and lives of women in early America. Ulrich has been quoted as saying that in her writing, she strives to show "the silent work of ordinary people." Ordinary, perhaps, but also profound.

Once More, with Gusto

Everyone—from you and your partner to grandparents, siblings (well, mostly), friends, coworkers, and even the neighbor at the corner who hauls your trash can to the curb when you forget—looks forward to the arrival of the new baby. It's a big and joyous event, and everyone wants to be part of it in some way. When you understand and accept the power you have within yourself to birth that baby, it's easy to look forward to the birthing with the same excitement and eagerness. You *know* you can do this. And you know that no matter what agenda your birth actually has, you'll have your best possible birth.

When you hold your new baby in your arms, you'll of course be thrilled and want to take in every molecule of his or her being. But how wonderful, too, to also think in the back of your mind, "I can't wait to do this again!"

The Least You Need to Know

- There are no secrets to having a happy, natural birth; every woman has all she needs right within herself already, right now.

- The power of birth touches everyone who stands in its energy.

- When you know what your body is capable of doing, you can look forward as much to your birthing experience as to the arrival of your baby.

- Knowing that you'll want to do this again may be the deciding factor for choosing natural birth the first time.

- All birth stories are beautiful stories.

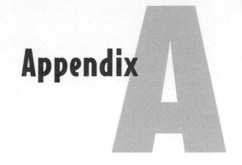
Resources

Books

Arms, Suzanne. *Immaculate Deception II: Myth, Magic, and Birth.* Berkeley, CA: Ten-Speed Press/Celestial Arts, 1994.

Bertram, Lakshmi. *Choosing Waterbirth: Reclaiming the Sacred Power of Birth.* Charlottesville, VA: Hampton Roads Publishing Company, 2000.

Block, Jennifer. *Pushed: The Painful Truth About Childbirth and Modern Maternity Care.* Cambridge, MA: Da Capo Press, 2007.

Bradley, Robert A., M.D. *Husband-Coached Childbirth, Fifth Edition.* New York: Bantam, 2008.

Buckley, Sarah J., M.D. *Gentle Birth, Gentle Mothering: A Doctor's Guide to Natural Childbirth and Gentle Early Parenting Choices.* Berkeley, CA: Ten-Speed Press/Celestial Arts, 2009.

Cortlund, Yana, Barb Lucke, and Donna Miller Watelet. *Mother Rising.* Berkeley, CA: Ten-Speed Press/Celestial Arts, 2006.

Davis, Elizabeth. *Heart & Hands: A Midwife's Guide to Pregnancy and Birth, Fourth Edition.* Berkeley, CA: Ten-Speed Press/Celestial Arts, 2004.

Declercq, E., C. Sakala, M. Corry, S. Applebaum, and P. Risher. *Listening to Mothers: Report of the First National U.S. Survey of Women's Childbearing Experiences.* New York: Maternity Center Association, 2002.

Declercq, E., C. Sakala, M. Corry, and S. Applebaum. *Listening to Mothers II: Report of the Second National U.S. Survey of Women's Childbearing Experiences.* New York: Childbirth Connection, 2006.

Dick-Read, Grantly. *Childbirth Without Fear: The Principles and Practice of Natural Childbirth.* London, England: Pinter & Martin, 2004.

Feldman, Gail Carr, and Eve Adamson. *Releasing the Mother Goddess.* Indianapolis: Alpha Books, 2003.

Fisher, Chloe, Suzanne Arms, and Mary Renfrew. *Bestfeeding: How to Breastfeed Your Baby, Third Edition.* Berkeley, CA: Ten-Speed Press/Celestial Arts, 2004.

Gaskin, Ina May. *Ina May's Guide to Childbirth.* New York: Bantam, 2003.

——— *Spiritual Midwifery, Fourth Edition.* Summertown, TN: Book Publishing Company, 2002.

Goer, Henci. *The Thinking Woman's Guide to a Better Birth.* New York: Penguin Group, 1999.

Harper, Barbara, R.N. *Gentle Birth Choices: A Guide to Making Informed Choices About Birthing Centers, Birth Attendants, Water Birth, Home Birth, and Hospital Birth.* Rochester, VT: Healing Arts Press, 2005.

Hawk, Breck, R.N. *Hey! Who's Having This Baby, Anyway? How to Take Charge and Create a Safe Environment for Your Baby's Birth, Including Essential Information About Medications and Interventions: A Guide and Workbook.* Yarnell, AZ: End Table Books, 2005.

Klaus, Marshall H., M.D., John H. Kennell, M.D., and Phyllis H. Klaus, CSW, MFT. *The Doula Book: How a Trained Labor Companion Can Help You Have a Shorter, Easier, and Healthier Birth.* Cambridge, MA: Perseus Publishing, 2002.

Klaus, Marshall H., M.D., and Phyllis H. Klaus, CSW, MFCC. *Your Amazing Newborn.* Cambridge, MA: Da Capo Press, 2000.

La Leche League International. *The Womanly Art of Breastfeeding, Seventh Revised Edition.* New York: Penguin Group, 2004.

Lipton, Bruce H., Ph.D. *The Biology of Belief: Unleashing the Power of Consciousness, Matter, and Miracles.* Mountain of Love Productions, 2008.

McCutcheon, Susan. *Natural Childbirth the Bradley Way.* New York: Plume, 1996.

Mongan, Marie F. *HypnoBirthing: The Mongan Method, A Natural Approach to a Safe, Easier, More Comfortable Birthing, Third Edition.* Deerfield Beach, FL: Health Communications, Inc., 2005.

Noble, Elizabeth. *Essential Exercises for the Childbearing Year: A Guide to Health and Comfort Before and After Your Baby Is Born, Fourth Edition.* Harwich, MA: New Life Images, 1995.

Odent, Michel. *Birth and Breastfeeding.* East Sussex, England: Clairview Books, 2003.

——— *The Caesarean.* London, England: Free Association Books, 2004.

Pryor, Gale, and Kathleen Huggins, R.N., M.S. *Nursing Mother, Working Mother.* Boston: The Harvard Common Press, 2007.

Sears, William, M.D., and Martha Sears, R.N. *The Baby Book: Everything You Need to Know About Your Child from Birth to Age Two, Revised and Updated.* New York: Little, Brown and Company, 2003.

Simpkin, Penny. *The Birth Partner: A Complete Guide to Childbirth for Dads, Doulas, and All Other Labor Companions, Third Edition.* Boston, MA: The Harvard Common Press, 2008.

Vincent, Peggy. *Baby Catcher: Chronicles of a Modern Midwife.* New York: Scribner, 2002.

Wagner, Marsden, M.D., M.S. *Born in the USA: How a Broken Maternity System Must Be Fixed to Put Women and Children First.* Berkeley, CA: University of California Press, 2008.

Wagner, Marsden, M.D., M.S., with Stephanie Gunning. *Creating Your Birth Plan: The Definitive Guide to a Safe and Empowering Birth.* New York: Penguin Group, 2006.

Wildner, Kim, CCE, CHT, HBCE. *Mother's Intention: How Belief Shapes Birth.* Ludington, MI: Harbor & Hill Publishing, 2003.

Wirth, Frederick. *Prenatal Parenting.* New York: HarperCollins, 2001.

Videos

Agaton, Mikael (writer, director, and producer). *The Miracle of Life* (DVD). NOVA/ WGBH Boston, 2000.

Grupper, Jonathan (director and producer). *From Conception to Birth* (DVD). The Discovery Channel, 2007.

Lake, Ricki (executive producer). *The Business of Being Born* (DVD). New Line Home Video, 2008.

MacDonald, Toby (writer and producer). *In the Womb* (DVD). National Geographic Video, 2006.

Townend, Lorne (writer and director). *In the Womb: Multiples* (DVD). National Geographic Video, 2006.

Websites

www.albuquerquehomebirth.com
The website of this book's midwife coauthor, Jennifer West, contains numerous articles and lots of information about natural birth and complementary methods including herbal teas and waterbirth.

www.birthingnaturally.net
This website offers comprehensive articles and information about natural childbirth with a section for Christian-specific approaches. The website's owner is childbirth educator and doula Jennifer VanderLaan, who has written several books and writes articles for other websites and publications.

www.bradleybirth.com
BradleyBirth.com is the website for the Bradley Method of natural childbirth. This site provides mostly information about how to find Bradley instructors and what's involved in the classes. Those who are registered for Bradley Method classes have access to a password-protected student resource center.

www.gentlebirth.org
California homebirth midwife Ronnie Falcao sponsors this website to provide information about homebirth (she has a separate website, linked from this one, for her midwifery services). The site features articles by Falcao as well as by other birthing experts. There are also study reports.

www.hypnobirthing.com
HypnoBirthing.com is the website of the Mongan Method of HypnoBirthing. This site contains information about HypnoBirthing, stories from parents about their birthing experiences, a directory of qualified practitioners, and an e-store.

www.waterbirth.org
Waterbirth.org is the website for Waterbirth International, a not-for-profit organization dedicated to making waterbirth possible for all women by bringing education, training, and supplies (including waterbirth tubs) to individuals, hospitals, and

birthing centers throughout the United States and around the world. Waterbirth International founder Barbara Harper, R.N., has dedicated her career to promoting the gentle birth of waterbirth. The website has numerous articles and research reports about waterbirth. Its e-store sells books, DVDs, birth pools, and related supplies.

Glossary

adrenaline   The body's "Let's go!" hormone, also called the fight-or-flight hormone. Another name for adrenaline is epinephrine.

amniotomy   The artificial rupture of the amniotic membranes ("breaking the water") using a hook-like device (amniotome) inserted into the vagina.

AROM   Common abbreviation for artificial rupture of membranes; see *amniotomy*.

board-certified specialty   An area of medical practice that requires several years of focused training after which the physician must pass written, oral, and skills examinations to receive board certification. Obstetrics is a board-certified specialty.

breech presentation   When the baby enters the birth path bottom first or feet first, rather than head first.

cesarean section   Surgical birth, commonly referred to as a c-section, in which the obstetrician makes incisions through the abdominal wall and the wall of the uterus to remove the baby.

complementary therapies   Methods or treatment approaches, sometimes called alternative medicine, that are outside the scope of conventional (allopathic) medicine.

conditioned response   A technique of gradually associating a stimulus with a desired response; also called classical conditioning or associative learning.

continuous electronic fetal monitoring (CEFM)   An ultrasound technology that transmits, displays, and records signals of uterine contractions and the baby's heart rate.

dilation   The size of the cervical opening. A fully dilated cervix is open to 10 centimeters.

direct-entry midwife   A midwife who has specific training and experience in birthing but is not a registered nurse (RN). A direct-entry midwife may or may not be certified and/or licensed.

diuretic   A substance that increases the body's excretion of fluid.

doula   A birth assistant who provides labor support such as personal care, comfort, encouragement, and advocacy during the birthing process but is not directly involved in the birth.

dystocia   A medical term that broadly means "abnormal birth." Doctors may use dystocia as a general description for labor that is not progressing as expected or specifically in association with the reason, such as shoulder dystocia (difficulty with the baby's shoulders making it through the birth path).

eclampsia   The advancement of preeclampsia into a potentially life-threatening condition in late pregnancy, the hallmarks of which are very high blood pressure (hypertension), extreme accumulation of fluid throughout the body (edema), protein in the urine, elevated liver enzymes, and often seizures.

effacement   The thinning and stretching of the cervix in preparation for birth, commonly expressed as a percentage with 100 percent being fully effaced.

en caul   Describes a baby born still fully enclosed in the unruptured amniotic membranes.

endorphins   Chemicals the body naturally produces and releases that act as potent pain relievers; a flood of endorphins may also have a euphoric effect.

epidural   A form of regional anesthesia in which an anesthetic agent is injected into the space around the spinal cord in the lower back. The effect is to numb sensation (including voluntary movement) in the lower part of the body. An "epidural lite" uses somewhat less medication to allow use of the legs.

episiotomy   A surgical incision through the tissues of the perineum to widen the vaginal opening.

evidence-based data   Measurable information collected about actual outcomes.

fetal Doppler   A device that uses ultrasound to detect the baby's heart tones before birth, to amplify the tones, and to project them as audible sounds.

fetoscope   A specialized stethoscope a practitioner uses to listen to the baby's heart tones; it has a platform that braces against the practitioner's forehead to use bone conduction to amplify the sounds so the practitioner can hear them.

GBS   Abbreviation for group-B streptococcus (strep), an infection commonly present in the vagina that can be harmful to the baby during birth if untreated. Testing for GBS in later pregnancy is standard.

gestational diabetes   The development of insulin resistance or diabetes during pregnancy, which usually corrects itself after birthing though may require insulin treatment until then.

half-life   The length of time it takes for the level of a drug in the body to be at half its original potency.

induced labor   The administration of synthetic oxytocin (Pitocin) to cause uterine contractions; also called induction.

lay midwife   A midwife who acquires her expertise through experience and assists with homebirths.

meconium   The tarlike substance that seals the baby's intestines before birth. The release of meconium during labor and before birth may be a sign that the baby is in distress, although about 10 percent of babies do this and only a small number of them are in distress.

meconium staining   The appearance of meconium in the amniotic fluid when the membranes rupture.

midwife   A nonphysician practitioner who is an expert in normal birth.

natural birth   Generally accepted to define a birth that takes place without medication or medical intervention.

nuchal   Means "around the neck." A nuchal cord occurs when the umbilical cord loops around the baby's neck; a nuchal hand occurs when the baby's hand is near its head at birth, with the hand and head emerging from the birth path at the same time.

nurse midwife   A registered nurse (RN) who has additional education and certification in midwifery.

oxytocin   A prostaglandin (hormone) the body naturally produces that has roles in love, sex, and birth. Oxytocin stimulates the contractions of labor.

physician assistant, certified (PA-C)   A medical practitioner who provides basic to mid-level medical care under the authority, although not necessarily direct supervision, of a physician.

Pitocin   Synthetic oxytocin; a drug administered to cause uterine contractions to induce labor, intensify labor that has slowed, or cause the uterus to "clamp down" after the placenta is out.

placenta abruptio   Detachment of the placenta from the wall of the uterus before birth.

placenta accreta   A placenta that grows more deeply than normal into the wall of the uterus, increasing the risk for difficulty of placental separation after birth as well as the potential for excessive blood loss.

placenta previa   A very low implantation of the placenta that may be near (marginal), encroach upon (moderate), or block (complete) the cervix.

prana   The Sanskrit word for "breath" that connotes life force or energy.

preeclampsia   The combination of high blood pressure, edema, and excess protein in the urine that may occur later in pregnancy.

prophylactic   A therapy or treatment, also called prophylaxis, intended to prevent something from happening.

puerperal fever   A serious bacterial infection that can develop in a woman following birth, when tissue trauma and cuts provide easy access for bacteria to enter the bloodstream.

relaxin   A hormone the placenta produces during pregnancy that causes connective tissue throughout the woman's body to soften and loosen, allowing increased flexibility of the joints.

standing orders   Prewritten instructions from a doctor or midwife that allow or direct the hospital or birthing center staff to take certain actions for all of a practitioner's patients upon admission to the facility.

transition   The final phase of labor's first stage, at which effort switches from preparing your body for birthing to the process of moving the baby along the birth path.

twilight sleep   A mix of the drugs scopolamine and morphine, administered intravenously to cause deep sedation.

universal precautions   The measures that health-care providers take to protect themselves from contact with bodily fluids.

VBAC   Vaginal birth after a previous cesarean birth; pronounced "VEE-back."

Index

A

A Midwife's Tale: The Life of Martha Ballard Based on Her Diary, 1785–1812, 289
abruptio (placenta abruptio), 72
accreta (placenta accreta), 71
ACOG (American College of Obstetrics and Gynecology), 97
active labor
    dealing with severe pain, 237-238
    overview, 220
    transition stage, 220-221
activities
    common activities, 56
    fitness considerations, 54-56
acupressure, 142-144
acupuncture, 142-143
adrenaline, overview, 46-47
Alade, Margaret, 274
alternate nostril breathing (yoga), 124-126
AMA (American Medical Association), 97
American College of Obstetrics and Gynecology. *See* ACOG
American Medical Association. *See* AMA
amniotomy, 16
anesthetized birth, 17
awareness, mindfulness techniques, 137

B

babies
    breastfeeding
        arrival of milk, 279
        bowel movement expectations, 280-281
        breast pumps, 280
        colostrum benefits, 278-279
        determining if baby is getting enough, 279-280
        IQ studies, 281
        lactation consultants, 275
        lifelong benefits, 281
        nursing shields, 277
        patience, 275-276
        positioning, 274-275
        root-latch-suck reflex, 274
        toughening nipples, 276-277
    doulas, 196-197
    fetal monitoring
        CEFM (continuous electronic fetal monitoring), 67
        fetal doppler, 68
        fetoscope, 68
    first moment considerations
        delayed cord clamping, 254
        first breath, 253-254
        skin-to-skin contact, 252-253
        smell, 255-256
    first twelve hour expectations, 255-259
        body dynamics, 256-257
        endorphin release, 258-259
        testing, 257-258
    formula-feeding, 278
    impact of birth process on, 51
    talking to, 259
baby blues versus postpartum depression, 266-269
Bach flower remedies, 144
Ballard, Martha, 289
basic breathing (yoga), 123
benefits
    colostrum, 278-279
    waterbirth, 173-174
bigness of birth, 232-233
birth-care providers
    doulas, 82-83
    interviewing, 86-91
    listing of providers, 78-79
    midwives, 79-82
        CNM (Certified Nurse Midwife), 80-81
        direct-entry midwives, 81-82
        lay midwives, 82
    physicians, 83-86
        board-certified specialty, 84
        family practitioners, 85-86
        obstetricians, 84-86
        PA (physician assistant), 84

selecting, 76-77
including support
partner in decision, 77
narrowing list, 77
birth energy, power of
author's experience, 286-287
secrets, 284-285
trust, 285-286
birth myths
homebirth, 7
hospital settings, 6
labor, 6-7
pain and misery, 6
pain medications, 7
birthing centers, 98
hospital-based, 100-101
midwifery birthing centers,
99-100
support members, 154
birthing experience
babies' first moments
delayed cord clamping,
254
first breath, 253-254
skin-to-skin contact,
252-253
smell, 255-256
birthing preferences
changing, 208
deal breakers, 207
documenting, 202-204
flexibility, 209
length, 206-207
stating your wants,
204-205
cesarean section, 22-23
childbirth education,
161-170
Bradley method, 166-167
core essentials, 162-163
costs, 164
finding classes, 168-170
homebirth, 168
HypnoBirthing, 167-168
instructors, 163-164

Lamaze method, 165-166
partner participation,
169-170
dangers
"do something"
syndrome, 67-69
eclampsia, 70
interventions, 66-67
mythology, 64-65
placenta problems, 71-72
preeclampsia, 70-71
statistical data, 65-66
versus scare tactics, 69-70
doulas
babies, 196-197
birth, 195-196
collaborating with, 200
hiring, 197-199
history, 192-193
independent, 199
modern, 193-194
postpartum, 196-197
qualifications, 197-198
roles and responsibilities,
194-195
staff, 199-200
evidence-based data, 20-21
first twelve hour
expectations (babies),
255-259
body dynamics, 256-257
endorphin release,
258-259
testing, 257-258
homebirth, 94
birth myths, 7
childbirth education, 168
children, 97
considering factors, 96
controversy, 97-98
pain medications, 7
statistics, 21
support members,
148-150
honoring the bigness of
birth, 232-233

hormones
adrenaline, 46-47
endorphins, 45-46
oxytocin, 44-45
hypnosis for birth, 182-190
believing in, 185
control issues, 186
evaluation studies,
188-189
history, 183
Hypnobabies, 187
HypnoBirthing, 187
misperceptions, 184
Natal Hypnotherapy, 187
New Way Childbirth,
187
Painless Childbirth
Program, 187
power of suggestion,
189-190
practicing, 185-186
process, 184-185
programs, 186-188
trance state, 183-184
impact on baby, 51
importance of birth story,
286-287
interventions
breech birth, 244-245
cesarean section, 19, 246
CPD (cephalopelvic
disproportion), 243-244
failure to progress, 243
laws and regulations, 20
meconium staining,
245-246
pain relief, 17-18
risks and benefits, 22
laboring down with
epidural, 242-243
labor process
active labor, 220-221
early labor, 216-219
first stage, 214
nonmedicated birth,
223-233

prelabor, 215-216
second stage, 214, 223-230
staying true to birth preferences, 221-222
third stage labor, 214, 230-231
making choices, 10-11
natural birth, 26
  commitments, 27-29
  dealing with opposition, 34
  defining characteristics, 14-16
  displaying confidence, 35
  history, 30-32
  overview, 13-14
  rewards, 29, 34
  risks, 32-33
orgasmic birth, 50-51
pain
  comfort measures, 48-50
  cultural origins, 40
  dealing with severe pain, 236-238
  labor experiences, 41-44
  medication intervention, 238-243
  power of expectation, 47-48
  worries and fears, 41-42
payment issues, 104-105
power of birth energy
  author's experience, 286-287
  secrets, 284-285
  trust, 285-286
power of language, 23-24
preparations, 9
reclaiming, 8-9
settings
  birthing centers, 98-101
  homebirth, 94-98
  hospitals, 101-104
  selection process, 94

stories
  importance, 286-287
  Nicole Kidman, 287-288
  overview, 4-5
  writing own story, 8
support members
  birthing centers, 154
  family, 155-157
  homebirth, 148-150
  hospital births, 150-154
  preparations, 157-158
  selection process, 148-149
talking to babies, 259
timing considerations, 21-22
waterbirth
  benefits, 173-174
  dive reflex in babies, 174-175
  effects on gravity, 172
  hospitals, 179-180
  tub considerations, 176-179
  water temperature, 176
  when to avoid, 175
blood pressure concerns
  eclampsia, 70
  preeclampsia, 70-71
BMI (body mass index), 59
board-certified specialty, 84
body considerations
  fitness
    body changes, 54
    common activities, 56
    nutrition, 59-60
    staying active, 54-56
    water workouts, 57
    weight, 58-59
    yoga, 57
  BMI (body mass index), 59
body mass index. *See* BMI
bowel movements, breastfeeding and, 280-281
Bradley method, 166-167

breaking of water, 217-218, 245-246
breastfeeding
  arrival of milk, 279
  bowel movement expectations, 280-281
  breast pumps, 280
  colostrum benefits, 278-279
  determining if baby is getting enough, 279-280
  IQ studies, 281
  lactation consultant, 275
  lifelong benefits, 281
  nursing shields, 277
  patience, 275-276
  positioning, 274-275
  root-latch-suck reflex, 274
  toughening nipples, 276-277
breast pumps, 280
breathing
  babies' first breath, 253-254
  yoga methods
    alternate nostril breathing, 124-126
    basic breathing, 123
    complete breathing, 123-124
    prana, 122
breech births, 244-245
Brewer Diet, 113
Business of Being Born, The, 98

C

calorie concerns (eating tips), 110-111
Cat Pose, 126
CEFM (continuous electronic fetal monitoring), 67
cephalopelvic disproportion. *See* CPD
Certified Nurse Midwife. *See* CNM
Certified Professional Midwife. *See* CPM

cervix
dilation, 48
effacement, 48
labor experience and pain, 43
cesarean section, 19-23
breech presentation, 244-245
CPD (cephalopelvic disproportion), 243-244
myths, 44
overview, 246
risks of natural birth, 33
changing birthing preferences, 208
childbirth education, 161-170
Bradley method, 166-167
core essentials, 162-163
costs, 164
finding classes, 168-170
homebirth, 168
HypnoBirthing, 167-168
instructors, 163-164
Lamaze method, 165-166
partner participation, 169-170
childbed fever, 30-31
children and homebirth, 97
classes, childbirth education, 168-170
CNM (Certified Nurse Midwife), 80-81
Cobbler's Pose, 126
colostrum, benefits, 278-279
comfort measures, 48-50
common methods, 49-50
hypnosis, 49
water, 49
commitments, 27-29
complementary therapies, 141
complete breathing (yoga), 123-124
complications (birth dangers)
"do something" syndrome, 67-69
eclampsia, 70

intervention, 66-67
mythology, 64-65
placenta problems
abruptio, 72
accreta, 71
previa, 72
preeclampsia, 70-71
statistical data, 65-66
versus scare tactics, 69-70
confidence, displaying, 35
continuous electronic fetal monitoring. *See* CEFM
controversies, homebirth, 97-98
cord clamping, 254
cortisol levels, lowering, 138-139
costs
childbirth education, 164
payment issues, 104-105
Cow Pose, 126
CPD (cephalopelvic disproportion), 243-244
CPM (Certified Professional Midwife), 81
CST (craniosacral therapy), 144
cultural origins, painful births, 40

D

dangers of birth
"do something" syndrome, 67-69
eclampsia, 70
intervention, 66-67
mythology, 64-65
placenta problems
abruptio, 72
accreta, 71
previa, 72
preeclampsia, 70-71
statistical data, 65-66
versus scare tactics, 69-70

deformities, skeletal, 31-32
delayed cord clamping, 254
depression (postpartum depression)
causes and treatments, 268
compounding factors, 268-269
versus baby blues, 266-268
diabetes (gestational), 58, 112-113
Dick-Read, Grantly (father of childbirth education), 48
diets, Brewer Diet, 113
dilation, 48
direct-entry midwives, 81-82
disagreements, handling family disagreements, 156-157
diuretics, 114
dive reflex, 174-175
documenting birthing preferences, 202-207
length, 206-207
stating your wants, 204-205
doppler (fetal), 68
"do something" syndrome, 67-69
doulas
as support members for hospital births, 153-154
baby, 196-197
birth, 195-196
collaborating with, 200
hiring, 197-199
history, 192-193
independent, 199
modern, 193-194
overview, 82-83
postpartum, 196-197
qualifications, 197-198
roles and responsibilities, 194-195
staff, 199-200
Downward-Facing Dog Pose, 126
drinking fluids, tips, 116-117
Duplicity, 288

E

early labor, 216
  breaking of water, 217-218
  dealing with pain, 237
  losing mucus plug, 217
  resting, 219
  whiny stage, 218-219
eating tips
  big babies, 112-113
  Brewer Diet, 113
  calories, 110-111
  fluid consumption, 116-117
  labor, 117-118
  morning sickness, 116
  natural foods, 116
  nutrition, 59-60
  postpartum considerations,
    263-264
  protein requirements,
    114-115
  weight, 111-112
eclampsia, 70
education (childbirth), 161-170
  Bradley method, 166-167
  core essentials, 162-163
  costs, 164
  finding classes, 168-170
  homebirth, 168
  HypnoBirthing, 167-168
  instructors, 163-164
  Lamaze method, 165-166
  partner participation,
    169-170
emotions, postpartum
  considerations, 263-264
en caul deliveries, 217
endorphins
  overview, 45-46
  release, 258-259
energy (birth energy),
  author's experience, 286-287
  secrets, 284-285
  trust, 285-286

energy therapies (mindfulness
  techniques), 141-144
  acupressure, 142-144
  "energy work," 144
epidural
  laboring down with, 242-243
  overview, 240-242
  pain intervention, 18
episiotomy, 16
*Everyday Blessings: The Inner
  Work of Mindful Parenting,*
  136
evidence-based data, 20-21
exercises, mindfulness
  techniques, 136

F

failure to progress, 243
family as support members
  asking for help, 157
  assigning roles, 155-156
  handling disagreements,
    156-157
family practitioners, selecting
  birth-care providers, 85-86
Farm Midwifery Center, 18
faucet extensions (birthing
  tubs), 177-179
fears and worries
  mindfulness techniques,
    137-138
  painful births, 41-42
fetal doppler, 68
fetal monitoring
  CEFM (continuous elec-
    tronic fetal monitoring),
    67
  fetal doppler, 68
  fetoscope, 68
fetoscope, 68
final preparations (homebirth),
  150
Firelog Pose, 126

first moments (babies)
  delayed cord clamping, 254
  first breath, 253-254
  skin-to-skin contact,
    252-253
  smell, 255-256
first stage labor, 214
first twelve hour expectations
  (babies), 255-259
  body dynamics, 256-257
  endorphin release, 258-259
  testing, 257-258
fish, mercury concerns, 115
fitness considerations
  body changes, 54
  common activities, 56
  nutrition, 59-60
  staying active, 54-56
  water workouts, 57
  weight, 58-59
  yoga, 57
flexibility (birthing
  preferences), 209
fluids, drinking tips, 116-117
foods, protein sources, 115
formula-feeding babies, 278

G

Gaskin, Ina May, 18
gestational diabetes, 58,
  112-113
Guinness Book of World Records,
  286

H

health conditions
  affects on pregnancy and
    birth, 60-61
  risks, 32, 61
Healthy People 2010, 278
heart rate monitoring
  CEFM (continuous elec-
    tronic fetal monitoring), 67

fetal doppler, 68
fetoscope, 68
hiring doulas, 197-199
history
  childbed fever, 30-31
  doulas, 192-193
  hypnosis for birth, 183
  skeletal deformities, 31-32
homebirth, 94
  birth myths, 7
  childbirth education, 168
  children, 97
  considering factors, 96
  controversies, 97-98
  pain medications, 7
  statistics, 21
  support members, 148-150
    final preparations, 150
    tasks and
      responsibilities, 149
hormones
  adrenaline, 46-47
  endorphins, 45-46
  oxytocin, 44-45
  postpartum considerations,
    262-263
  relaxin, 120-121
hospital-based birthing
  centers, 100-101
hospital births
  as setting for natural birth,
    101-104
    business aspects, 102-103
    safeguarding natural
      birth options, 103-104
  birthing tubs, 179-180
  support members, 150-154
    claiming your space,
      151-152
    dealing with protocols
      and routines, 152-153
    doulas, 153-154
Howell, Maggie, Natal
  Hypnotherapy, 187
Hypnobabies, 187

HypnoBirthing (Mongan
  Method), 167-168, 187
hypnosis for birth, 49, 182
  believing in, 185
  control issues, 186
  evaluation studies, 188-189
  history, 183
  Hypnobabies, 187
  HypnoBirthing, 187
  misperceptions, 184
  Natal Hypnotherapy, 187
  New Way Childbirth, 187
  Painless Childbirth
    Program, 187
  power of suggestion,
    189-190
  practicing, 185-186
  process, 184-185
  programs, 186, 188
    Hypnobabies, 187
    HypnoBirthing, 187
    instructor qualifications,
      187-188
    Natal Hypnotherapy, 187
    New Way Childbirth,
      187
    Painless Childbirth
      Program, 187
    partner participation, 188
  trance state, 183-184

I–J

independent doulas, 199
infections, childbed fever, 30-31
instructors
  childbirth education,
    163-164
  hypnosis programs, 187-188
insurance coverage, 104-105
integrative care, 85
intervention
  birth dangers, 66-70
  breech birth, 244-245
  cesarean section, 19-23, 246

CPD (cephalopelvic
  disproportion), 243-244
failure to progress, 243
laws and regulations, 20
meconium staining, 245-246
medication intervention,
  238-243
  epidural, 240-243
  narcotics, 239-240
pain relief
  anesthetized birth, 17
  epidural, 18
  "twilight sleep," 18
risks and benefits, 22
interviewing health-care
  providers, 86-91
IQ studies, breastfeeding, 281

K–L

Kabat-Zinn, Jon, 136
Kein, Gerald, Painless
  Childbirth Program, 187
Kidman, Nicole, birth story,
  287-288
labor process
  active labor
    overview, 220
    transition, 220-221
  birth myths, 6-7
  doulas
    birth, 195-196
    history, 192-193
    modern, 193-194
    roles and responsibilities,
      194-195
  early labor, 216-219
    breaking of water,
      217-218
    losing mucus plug, 217
    resting, 219
    whiny stage, 218-219
  eating tips, 117-118
  first stage, 214

hypnosis for birth, 182-190
  believing in, 185
  control issues, 186
  evaluation studies, 188-189
  history, 183
  Hypnobabies, 187
  HypnoBirthing, 187
  misperception, 184
  Natal Hypnotherapy, 187
  New Way Childbirth, 187
  Painless Childbirth Program, 187
  power of suggestion, 189-190
  practicing, 185-186
  process, 184-185
  programs, 186-188
  trance state, 183-184
impact on baby, 51
intervention
  breech birth, 244-245
  cesarean section, 246
  CPD (cephalopelvic disproportion), 243-244
  failure to progress, 243
  meconium staining, 245-246
laboring down with epidural, 242-243
massage, 133
nonmedicated birth, 223-233
  essence of time, 225-226
  honoring the bigness of birth, 232-233
  pushing stage, 227-230
  second stage, 223-227
  third stage labor, 230-231
  tuning in to inner messages, 225
  wait-and-save dynamic, 226-227
orgasmic birth, 50-51

pain, 41-42
  cervix, 43
  comfort measures, 48-50
  dealing with severe pain, 236-238
  power of expectation, 47-48
  medication intervention, 238-243
  surgical birth myths, 44
prelabor, 215-216
  nesting, 215
  practice labor, 215
second stage, 214, 223-230
  essence of time, 225-226
  pushing stage, 227-230
  tuning in to inner messages, 225
  wait-and-save dynamic, 226-227
staying true to birth preferences, 221-222
stretching techniques, 130-131
third stage, 214
third stage labor, 214, 230-231
waterbirth
  benefits, 173-174
  dive reflex in babies, 174-175
  effects on gravity, 172
  hospitals, 179-180
  tubs, 176-179
  water temperature, 176
  when to avoid, 175
yoga, 127-128
lactation consultants, 275
Lamaze method, 165-166
language, power of, 23-24
laws and regulations, 20
lay midwives, 82
lifelong benefits of breastfeeding, 281

Lion Pose, 127
Long, Crawford, 17

M

massage techniques, 131-133
  labor process, 133
  perineal massage, 132-133
  self-massage, 132
meconium staining intervention, 245-246
medication intervention, 238-243
  epidural, 240-243
  narcotics, 239-240
midwifery birthing centers, 99-100
midwives, 79-82
  CNM (Certified Nurse Midwife), 80-81
  direct-entry midwives, 81-82
  lay midwives, 82
mindfulness techniques
  awareness to present moment, 137
  energy therapies, 141-144
    acupressure, 142-144
    "energy work," 144
  lowering cortisol levels, 138-139
  mind over matter concept, 139-141
  overcoming fears and worries, 137-138
  practice exercise, 136
Mongan Method (Hypno-Birthing), 167-168, 187
monitoring
  CEFM (continuous electronic fetal monitoring), 67
  fetal doppler, 68
  fetoscope, 68
morbidity, 40

morning sickness, eating tips, 116
mortality, 40
mucus plug, 217
multiples, risks, 33
myths
cesarean section, 44
homebirth, 7
hospital settings, 6
labor, 6-7
pain and misery, 6
pain medications, 7

N

narcotic medications, 239-240
NARM (North American Registry of Midwives), 81
Natal Hypnotherapy, 187
natural birth, 26
commitments, 27-29
dealing with opposition, 34
defining characteristics, 14-16
displaying confidence, 35
evidence-based data, 20-21
history
childbed fever, 30-31
skeletal deformities, 31-32
homebirth, 21
hormones
adrenaline, 46-47
endorphins, 45-46
oxytocin, 44-45
impact on baby, 51
intervention, 22
orgasmic birth, 50-51
overview, 13-14
pain
comfort measures, 48-50
labor experiences, 41-44
power of expectation, 47-48
payment issues, 104-105

power of language, 23-24
rewards, 29, 34
risks
health conditions, 32
multiples, 33
previous cesarean sections, 33
settings
birthing centers, 98-101
homebirth, 94-98
hospitals, 101-104
selection process, 94
timing considerations, 21-22
natural foods, eating tips, 116
nesting, 215
New Way Childbirth, 187
nipples
nursing shields, 277
toughening, 276-277
nonmedicated birth
essence of time, 225-226
honoring the bigness of birth, 232-233
pushing stage
following bodily urges, 227-229
steady pushes, 229-230
second stage labor, 223-227
third stage labor, 230-231
tuning in to inner messages, 225
wait-and-save dynamic, 226-227
North American Registry of Midwives. *See* NARM
nutrition
eating tips, 59-60
big babies, 112-113
Brewer Diet, 113
calories, 110-111
labor, 117-118
morning sickness, 116
natural foods, 116

protein requirements, 114-115
weight, 111-112
fluid consumption, 116-117

O

obstetricians, selecting birth-care providers, 84-86
opposition, dealing with, 34
orders (standing orders), 67
orgasmic birth, 50-51
oxytocin, 44-45

P

PA (physician assistant), 84
packing considerations, 154-155
pain
comfort measures, 48-50
common methods, 49-50
hypnosis, 49
water, 49
cultural origins, 40
dealing with severe pain, 236-238
active labor, 237-238
early labor, 237
intervention
anesthetized birth, 17
epidural, 18
"twilight sleep," 18
labor experiences, 41-44
cervix, 43
surgical birth myths, 44
medication intervention, 238-243
epidural, 240-243
narcotics, 239-240
nonmedicated birth
essence of time, 225-226
honoring the bigness of birth, 232-233
pushing stage, 227-230

second stage labor, 223-227

third stage labor, 230-231

tuning in to inner messages, 225

wait-and-save dynamic, 226-227

power of expectation

positive thinking tips, 47-48

remaining calm, 48

worries and fears, 41-42

Painless Childbirth Program, 187

partner participation

childbirth education, 169-170

hypnosis programs, 188

payment issues, 104-105

perineal massage, 132-133

physician assistant. *See* PA

physicians, selecting birth-care providers, 83-86

board-certified specialty, 84

family practitioners, 85-86

obstetricians, 84-86

PA (physician assistant), 84

Pigeon Pose, 127

placenta

birth dangers

abruptio, 72

accreta, 71

previa, 72

delivery, 230-231

poses (yoga), 125-127

Cat Pose, 126

Cobbler's Pose, 126

Cow Pose, 126

Downward-Facing Dog Pose, 126

Firelog Pose, 126

Lion Pose, 127

Pigeon Pose, 127

Side Plank Pose, 127

Staff Pose, 127

Tiger Pose, 127

Triangle Pose, 127

Warrior Poses, 127

positioning, breastfeeding, 274-275

postpartum considerations

dealing with visitors, 265

doulas, 196-197

eating tips, 263-264

emotional issues, 263-264

hormonal shifts, 262-263

pacing yourself, 266

postpartum depression

causes and treatments, 268

compounding factors, 268-269

versus baby blues, 266-268

sexual intercourse, 269-271

support members, 264-265

two-week milestones, 266-267

practice labor, 215

prana, 122

preeclampsia, 70-71

preferences (birthing preferences)

changing, 208

deal breakers, 207

documenting, 202-204

flexibility, 209

length, 206-207

stating your wants, 204-205

prelabor, 215-216

nesting, 215

practice labor, 215

preparations, 9

birthing preferences

changing, 208

deal breakers, 207

documenting, 202-204

flexibility, 209

length, 206-207

stating your wants, 204-205

homebirth, 150

selecting support members, 157-158

previa (placenta previa), 72

programs (hypnosis for birth), 186-188

Hypnobabies, 187

HypnoBirthing, 187

instructor qualifications, 187-188

Natal Hypnotherapy, 187

New Way Childbirth, 187

Painless Childbirth Program, 187

partner participation, 188

protein, eating tips, 114-115

protocols, dealing with hospital protocols, 152-153

providers (birth-care)

doulas, 82-83

interviewing, 86-91

listing of providers, 78-79

midwives, 79-82

CNM (Certified Nurse Midwife), 80-81

direct-entry midwives, 81-82

lay midwives, 82

physicians, 83-86

board-certified specialty, 84

family practitioners, 85-86

obstetricians, 84-86

PA (physician assistant), 84

selecting, 76-77

including support partner in decision, 77

narrowing list, 77

puerperal fever, 30-31

pumps (breast), 280
pushing stage
    following bodily urges,
        227-229
    steady pushes, 229-230

Q-R

Qi Gong, 144
QT (Quantum Touch), 144
qualifications, doulas, 197-198
Quantum Touch. *See* QT

reclaiming birth, 8-9
Reiki, 144
relaxation methods
    massage, 131-133
        labor process, 133
        perineal massage, 132-133
        self-massage, 132
    stretching
        labor process, 130-131
        routines, 128-129
        swim strokes, 129-130
    yoga, 121-128
        breathing, 122-126
        labor process, 127-128
        poses, 125-127
relaxin, 120-121
rewards, 29, 34
Righard, Lennart, 274
risks
    health, 61
    natural birth
        health conditions, 32
        multiples, 33
        previous cesarean
            sections, 33
roles and responsibilities
    doulas, 194-195
    support members, 149
root-latch-suck reflex
    (breastfeeding), 274

routines, stretching, 128-129
rupture of membranes, 217-218

S

second stage labor, 214, 223-230
    essence of time, 225-226
    pushing stage
        following bodily urges,
            227-229
        steady pushes, 229-230
    tuning in to inner messages,
        225
    wait-and-save dynamic,
        226-227
selection process
    birth-care providers, 76-91
        doulas, 82-83
        including support
            partner in decision, 77
        interview process, 86-91
        listing of providers, 78-79
        midwives, 79-82
        narrowing list, 77
        physicians, 83-86
    birth settings
        birthing centers, 98-101
        homebirth, 94-98
        hospitals, 101-104
    support members
        birthing centers, 154
        family, 155-157
        homebirth, 148-150
        hospital births, 150-154
        preparations, 157-158
self-massage, 132
settings
    birthing centers, 98-101
        hospital-based, 100-101
        midwifery birthing
            centers, 99-100
    homebirth, 94-98
        children, 97
        considering factors, 96
        controversy, 97-98

hospitals, 101-104
    business aspects, 102-103
    safeguarding natural
        birth options, 103-104
    selection process, 94
sexual intercourse, postpartum,
    269-271
shields (nursing), 277
showers versus birthing tubs,
    179
Side Plank Pose, 127
skeletal deformities, 31-32
skin-to-skin contact, 252-253
smell, bonding with baby,
    255-256
staff doulas, 199-200
Staff Pose, 127
standing orders, 67
statistical data, birth dangers,
    65-66
stories (birth)
    importance, 286-287
    Nicole Kidman, 287-288
    overview, 4-5
    writing own story, 8
stress, cortisol levels, 138-139
stretching
    labor process, 130-131
    routines, 128-129
    swim strokes, 129-130
support members
    birthing centers, 154
    childbirth education,
        169-170
    dealing with opposition, 34
    family
        asking for help, 157
        assigning roles, 155-156
        handling disagreements,
            156-157
    homebirth, 148-150
        final preparations, 150
        tasks and responsibilities,
            149

hospital births, 150-154
  claiming your space,
    151-152
  dealing with protocols
    and routines, 152-153
  doulas, 153-154
  packing considerations,
    154-155
  postpartum considerations,
    264-265
  preparations, 157-158
  selection process, 148-149
swim strokes, stretching
  techniques, 129-130

T

talking to babies, 259
TBM (Total Body Modifica-
  tion), 144
testing babies, 257-258
Therapeutic Touch. *See* TT
third stage labor, 214, 230-231
three-part breathing (yoga),
  123-124
Tiger Pose, 127
Total Body Modification. *See*
  TBM
toughening nipples, 276-277
trance state (hypnosis for
  birth), 183-184
transition, 46, 220-221
treatments, postpartum
  depression, 268
Triangle Pose, 127
trusting yourself, 285-286
TT (Therapeutic Touch), 144
tubs (birthing)
  considering factors, 176-179
    faucet extensions, 177-179
    regular bathtubs, 178-179
    showers, 179
  hospitals, 179-180

Tuschhoff, Kerry,
  Hypnobabies, 187
"twilight sleep," 18
twins, risks, 33
two-week milestones
  (postpartum), 266-267

U-V

Ulrich, Laurel Thatcher, 289
universal precautions, 180

vaginal birth after cesarean
  section. *See* VBAC
Vassilyev, Feodor, 286
VBAC (vaginal birth after
  cesarean section), 23
visitors, postpartum
  considerations, 265

W-X

wait-and-save dynamic (nonmedicated birth), 226-227
Warrior Poses, 127
water
  as comfort measure, 49
  breaking of water, 217-218,
    245-246
  drinking requirements,
    116-117
  workouts, 57
waterbirth
  benefits, 173-174
  dive reflex in babies, 174-175
  effects on gravity, 172
  tub considerations, 176-180
    faucet extensions, 177-179
    hospitals, 179-180
    regular bathtubs, 178-179
    showers, 179
  water temperature, 176
  when to avoid, 175

websites
  Hypnobabies, 187
  New Way Childbirth, 187
  Omnihypnosis, 187
weight concerns
  BMI (body mass index), 59
  eating tips, 111-112
  fitness considerations, 58-59
whiny stage, 218-219
worries
  mindfulness techniques,
    137-138
  painful births, 41-42

Y-Z

yoga, 121
  breathing
    alternate nostril
      breathing, 124-126
    basic breathing, 123
    complete breathing,
      123-124
    prana, 122
  labor process, 127-128
  overview, 57
  poses, 125-127
    Cat Pose, 126
    Cobbler's Pose, 126
    Cow Pose, 126
    Downward-Facing Dog
      Pose, 126
    Firelog Pose, 126
    Lion Pose, 127
    Pigeon Pose, 127
    Side Plank Pose, 127
    Staff Pose, 127
    Tiger Pose, 127
    Triangle Pose, 127
    Warrior Poses, 127

Babies don't come with owners' manuals. You need *The Complete Idiot's Guides*®!

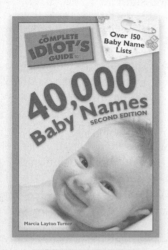
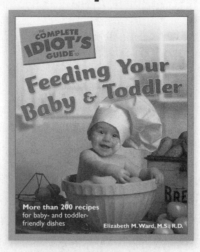
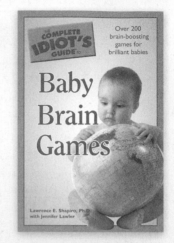
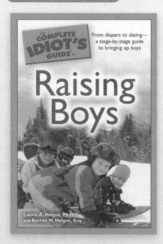
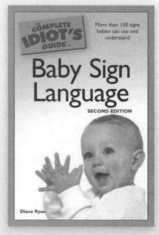
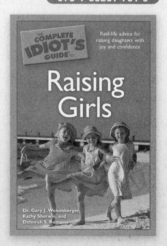
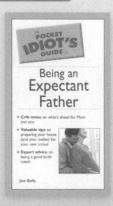
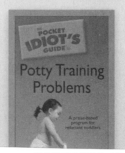
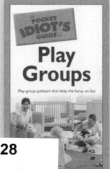
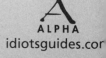
31901050485228